5 MINUTE PSYCHOTHERAPY TECHNIQUES

TRAUMA-INFORMED PRACTICES

JENNY H. HSUEH, MD

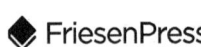

One Printers Way
Altona, MB R0G 0B0
Canada

www.friesenpress.com

Copyright © 2024 by Jenny H. Hsueh
First Edition — 2024

All rights reserved.

No part of this publication may be reproduced in any form, or by any means, electronic or mechanical, including photocopying, recording, or any information browsing, storage, or retrieval system, without permission in writing from FriesenPress.

ISBN
978-1-03-919300-0 (Hardcover)
978-1-03-919299-7 (Paperback)
978-1-03-919301-7 (eBook)

1. PSYCHOLOGY, PSYCHOTHERAPY, COUNSELING

Distributed to the trade by The Ingram Book Company

Contents

Foreword by Harry Zeit, MD 13
Prologue 15
Part I: Techniques 19
Chapter 1: Mindfulness and Body Techniques . . . 20
Mind-Body Connection 20

Stage 1 Skills 21
Technique #1: Slow Outbreath 21
Technique #2: Orienting to the Present 22
Technique #3: Engaging the Five Senses 23
Technique #4: One Mindful Thing 24
Technique #5: Exercise 25
Technique #6: Mindful Movements 26
Technique #7: Progressive Muscle Relaxation 26
Technique #8: Tapping / Emotional Freedom Technique 28
Technique #9: Diver's Reflex 29
Technique #10: Balancing on Uneven Ground 30
Technique #11: Dual Awareness with Hands 30
Technique #12: Observing Without Words 31
Technique #13: Mindful Check-in 32
Technique #14: Changing Body Position to Change Sensation 32

Stage 2 Skills 33
Technique #14: Variation A: Exaggerating Body Posture to Heighten Sensation . . . 33
Technique #15: Mindfulness about Absentmindedness 34
Technique #16: Mindfulness about Autopilot Mode 34
Technique #17: Mindfulness about Being Present and Being Absentminded . . . 35
Technique #18: Mindful Action with Traumatic Memory 35

Summary 36

Chapter 2: Metacognition / Mentalizing 37
State of Mind 38
Stage 1 Skills 38
Technique #1: Teaching Language for Emotions 38
Technique #2: Addressing Fears and Myths about Emotions 39
Technique #3: Window of Tolerance / Identifying the Intensity of Emotions 40
Technique #4: Judgments Versus Facts 41
Technique #5: Creating Distance with Mentalizing. 42
Technique #6: Identifying States of Mind, Balanced Perspectives 42
Technique #7: Using Scale for Awareness 43
Technique #8: Therapist Attunement for Awareness 44
Technique #9: Reflecting on Behaviour 44
Technique #10: Curiosity and "I Wonder" Statements 45
Technique #11: Pros and Cons 46
Technique #12: Journaling 47
Stage 2 Skills 47
Technique #13: Observing Emotions 47
Technique #14: Bringing Awareness to Self 47
Summary 49

Chapter 3: Fostering Positive Experiences 50
Stage 1 Skills 51
Technique #1: Self-Care. 51
Technique #2: Addressing Vulnerabilities 51
Technique #3: Positive Activities 52
Technique #4: Reframing 52
Technique #5: Happiness and Positives 54
Technique #6: Self-Compassion 55
Technique #7: Values 56
Technique #8: Setting Boundaries 56
Technique #9: Setting Goals 56
Technique #10: Problem Solving 57
Technique #11: Mastery and Competence 58
Technique #12: Self-Esteem 59
Technique #13: Fostering Hope and Optimism 60
Technique #14: Finding Meaning. 60

Technique #15: Building Resilience 61
Technique #16: Combining Techniques from Chapters 1 and 3 61
Technique #17: Combining Techniques from Chapters 2 and 3 62

Stage 2 Skills 62
Technique #18: Rewriting Your Story and Reframing 62
Technique #19: Self-Forgiveness 63
Technique #20: Forgiving Others 64

Summary 64

Chapter 4: Using Imagination / Hypnotic Techniques   65

Stage 1 Skills 66
Technique #1: Imagining a Safe Place 66
Technique #2: Imagining a Personal Bubble 67
Technique #3: Mood Dial 67
Technique #4: Chronic Pain Management Techniques 68
Technique #5: Imagining Cleansing 69
Technique #6: Auto-hypnosis using a Mirror 69
Technique #7: Shrinking Negative Emotions 70
Technique #8: Imagining Success 70
Technique #9: Healing the Inner Child 71

Stage 2 Skills 74
Technique #9: Variation B: Letter to Inner Child 74
Technique #10: Imagining an Ideal Partner 75
Technique #11: Working with Nightmares 76
Technique #12: Funeral of Broken Dreams 77
Technique #13: Imagining a Timeline with Positive Experiences 77

Working with Traumatic Memories 78
Technique #14: Boxing Difficult Memories 78
Technique #15: Screens Method 79
Technique #16: Adding Imaginary Elements 79

Summary 80

Chapter 5: Cognitive Behavioural Therapy (CBT) . . 81
The ABCs of CBT 81
Anxiety Model 82
Cognitive Dissonance 84

Stage 1 Skills 84

Cognition 84
Technique #1: Cognitive Distortions / Hot Thoughts 84
Technique #2: Therapist to Identify and Challenge Hot Thoughts 86
Technique #3: Myths About Thoughts 88
Technique #4: Creating Distance from Hot Thoughts 89
Technique #5: Antecedent, Belief, Consequence 89
Technique #6: Getting to the Core Belief 90
Technique #7: Facts Supporting, Facts Against 91
Technique #8: Locus of Control 91
Technique #9: Assigning Responsibility 92
Technique #10: Cumulative Probability 92

Affect 93
Technique #11: Noticing the Emotion and Situation 93
Technique #12: Adding Body Sensation 94

Behaviour 94
Technique #13: Antecedent, Behaviour, Consequence 94
Technique #14: Rewarding Desired Behaviour 95
Technique #15: Behaviour Activation 96

Combined 97
Technique #16: Putting it Together 97
Technique #17: Ambivalence / Working with Parts 98
Technique #18: Working with the Self-Critical Part 99

Stage 2 Skills 100

Exposure Treatment: 100
Technique #19: Story on Fear and Avoidance 100
Technique #20: Exposure Treatment 100
Technique #21: Meaning of the Exposure Treatment 102
Technique #22: Combining Exposure Treatment with Mindfulness 102

Summary 103

Chapter 6: Interpersonal Therapy (IPT) 104
Goals of IPT 104
Society and Culture. 105
Ingredients: 105
Consideration 106

Stage 1 Skills. 106

Information Gathering 106
Technique #1: Exploring Patients' Social Networks 106
Technique #2: Closeness Circle 107
Technique #3: How has the Relationship Changed. 108
Technique #4: Self-Awareness 109

Identifying Issues 109
Technique #5: Exploring the Issue 109
Technique #6: Exploring Expectations 110

Communication 110
Technique #7: Turn-Taking / Speaker Object 110
Technique #8: "I" Statement. 111
Technique #9: Beyond What is Said 111
Technique #10: Active Listening 112
Technique #11: Practicing Self-Disclosures and Small Favours. 112
Technique #12: Giving Feedback. 113

Emotional Regulation. 114
Technique #13: Self-Check-in Before and During Communication 114
Technique #14: Planning Ahead 114
Technique #15: Writing as Communication 115
Technique #16: Acknowledging Emotions. 115
Technique #17: De-escalation Skills 116

Problem Solve and Negotiate 116
Technique #18: Knowing Yourself 116
Technique #19: Patients Gathering Information 117
Technique #20: Reframing Unhelpful Thoughts 117
Technique #21: Exploring Strategies 118
Technique #22: Focusing on the Problem not the Person 119
Technique #23: Positive Associations / Create Opportunistic Times 120

Technique #24: Order of Requests 120
Technique #25: Researching Options. 120
Technique #26: Rewarding Good Behaviours 121
Technique #27: Therapist Role-Playing 121
Technique #28: Ending the Relationship 122

Stage 2 Skills 122
Technique #29: Grief 122

Summary 123

Chapter 7: Dialectical Behaviour Therapy (DBT) / Beyond the Classic CBT 124

Stage 1 Skills 125
Technique #1: Radical Acceptance 125
Technique #2: STOP Skill 125
Technique #3: Opposite Action 126

Stage 2 Skills 127
ABCs of CBT for Trauma (Build on Chapter 5 Skills) 127

Changing Trauma-Related Emotions. 129
Technique #4: Anger 129
Technique #5: Disgust 130
Technique #6: Fear 131
Technique #7: Guilt 132
Technique #8: Shame and Self-Blame 133
Technique #9: Mixed Emotions 135

Changing Trauma-Related Beliefs. 136
Technique #10: Identifying Trauma-Related Beliefs 136
Technique #11: Hot Thoughts in Context of Trauma 140
Technique #12: CBT Recording for Trauma 140
Technique #13: Challenging Trauma-Related Beliefs 141
Technique #14: Assigning Responsibility to Trauma 142
Technique #15: Role-Playing Friend 142
Technique #16: Going into Trauma Details 143
Technique #17: Narrative Exposure 143
Technique #18: Staying Grounded while Processing Traumatic Memory. . . 145
Technique #19: Challenging the Meaning of Traumatic Events 145

Technique #20: Birthday Speech. 146
Technique #21: Future Orientation and Focusing on Positives 147

Changing Trauma-Related Behaviour 148
Technique #22: Mindfulness of Craving 148
Technique #23: ACT. 148

Summary 149

Part II: Applications 151

Chapter 8: Attachment and the Therapeutic Relationship 152
Knowledge #1: Attachments. 153
Knowledge #2: Understanding "Challenging Patients" Through Attachment and Countertransference 159
Knowledge #3: Traumatic Re-enactment 160
Knowledge #4: Limiting Therapist Self-Disclosure. 161
Knowledge #5: Therapist Stance for Trauma-Informed Care 161

Structure Therapy 163
Technique #1: Identifying Patient Baseline 163
Technique #2: Setting Expectations 163
Technique #3: Sample Contract 164
Technique #4: Connection 166
Technique #5: Priorities and Aligning Goals / Getting Buy-in 166
Technique #6: Therapy-Disrupting Behaviour 167
Technique #7: Maintaining Boundaries 168
Technique #8: Safety 168
Technique #9: Slowing Down the Process 169
Technique #10: Choice 169
Technique #11: Curious 170
Technique #12: Validation 170
Technique #13: Balancing between Validation and Challenge 171
Technique #14: Secrecy and Truth Telling. 172
Technique #15: Resistance 173
Technique #16: Contradicting Behaviour 174
Technique #17: Avoidance 174
Technique #18: Exploring Fears About the Relationship 175

Addressing Traumatic Re-enactment 176
Knowledge #6: Step 1 Therapist Mentalizing 176
Knowledge #7: Step 2 Discussing the Relationship 177
Knowledge #8: Step 3 Repairing the Relationship 178
Technique #20: Addressing Misinterpretations 178
Technique #21: Therapist as Perpetrator 179
Technique #22: Therapist as Victim 180
Technique #23: Therapist as Rescuer 181
Technique #24: Therapist as Bystander 182

Summary 183

Chapter 9: Psychological Trauma 184
Knowledge #1: What is Trauma 184
Knowledge #2: Multigenerational Trauma 185
Knowledge #3: Adverse Childhood Experiences (ACEs) 185
Knowledge #4: Positive Childhood Experiences 186
Knowledge #5: Toxic Stress / Chronic Stress 186
Knowledge #6: Moral Injury 187
Knowledge #7: PTSD 187
Knowledge #8: Developmental Trauma Disorder (DTD) 188
Knowledge #9: Complex Trauma (CT) 189
Knowledge #10: Pathological Self-Soothing / Addiction 190
Knowledge #11: Dissociation 191
Knowledge #12: Trauma's Impact on Physical Body and Disease 191
Knowledge #13: Somatoform Dissociation 192
Knowledge #14: When to Consider DTD and CT 193
Knowledge #15: Defence Responses 194
Technique #1: Taking a Trauma History 198
Technique #2: Psychoeducation 199
Technique #3: Psychoeducation on Triggers 200
Technique #4: Working with Triggers 201
Technique #5: Working with the Fight Response 202
Technique #6: Working with the Flight Response 202
Technique #7: Working with the Freeze Response 203
Technique #8: Working with the Faint Response 204
Technique #9: Working with the Fawn Response 204
Technique #10: Working with the Attach Response 205

Stepwise Treatment 206
Knowledge #16: Step 1 Stabilizing 206
Knowledge #17: Step 2 Processing Memory 207
Knowledge #18: Step 3 Post-traumatic Growth / New Normal 209

Summary 211

Chapter 10: Clinical Cases 212

Clinical Cases 212

Dysregulated Mood 214
Case #1: Labile Mood in Late Life 214
Case #2: Grief and End of Life 217
Case #3: Postpartum Depression 220
Case #4: Teenager with Depression 224
Case #5: Child with Anxiety 227

Dysregulated Physiology 229
Case #6: Senior with Insomnia 229
Case #7: Functional Abdominal Pain 234

Dysregulated Behaviour 237
Case #8: Teenager with Eating Disorder 237
Case #9: Teenager with Obsessive Compulsive Disorder (OCD) 241
Case #10: Hoarding 243
Case #11: Substance Abuse 244

Dysregulated Self and Relationship 249
Case #12: Borderline Personality Disorder 249

PTSD / Simple Trauma 252
Case #13: Acute Stress in a Refugee 252
Case #14: Dog Attack 255

Dissociation 259
Case #15: Dissociation and Peripartum Mental Health 259

Complex Trauma 263
Case #16: Complex PTSD in a Veteran 263
Case #17: Dissociative Identity Disorder (DID) 268

Special Populations 274

Therapist Wellness and Peak Performance	275
Summary	277
Conclusion	278
Acknowledgements	279
Bibliography	280
Acronym Index	286

FOREWORD BY HARRY ZEIT, MD

Our era of prolonged distress and uncertainty has imposed unprecedented levels of stress on family physicians. There have been increasingly urgent calls to adopt trauma-informed care approaches to support the well-being of both primary care physicians and those in their care. But, for many, the term remains ill-defined and difficult to apply.

Alongside this, an increasing number of patients are presenting to family practitioners' offices with mental health issues or comorbidity and cannot afford private psychotherapy or the long waits for psychiatric consultation.

Accessible and practical, Dr. Hsueh's book presents a treasure trove of trauma-informed psychotherapy interventions and tools from a wide variety of models and approaches. Many of them can readily be integrated into regular office visits. This generous and diverse collection of interventions captures the spirit of trauma-informed mental health care, offering a multitude of techniques that can be applied immediately or utilized as a foundation for deeper exploration with fellow clinicians.

A rich assortment of case examples, well-known to every primary care provider, flesh out this gem of a book. This is not a preachy book or a political book; it's all about boots on the ground and using these skills right now to make an impact on our own distress and the distress of those in our care. It speaks to meeting the needs of our most complex and challenging patients.

With the potential to reduce physician and patient emotional suffering and to promote trauma awareness, I highly recommend that

Five Minute Psychotherapy Techniques: Trauma-Informed Practices be kept close at hand in every family medicine clinic and office.

Harry Zeit, MD, MDPAC(C), Certified in Sensorimotor Psychotherapy, former American Board-Certified Emergency Physician, founder of the Caring for Self while Caring for Others program.

PROLOGUE

This book is a one-stop resource that makes psychotherapy from a variety of schools of thought easy to learn and apply. The techniques are trauma-informed, evidence-based, and drawn from mindfulness, body-based therapy, cognitive behavioural therapy, mentalization-based therapy, interpersonal therapy, dialectical behaviour therapy, psychoanalysis, and hypnotherapy.

The techniques are versatile. They can be used to treat many different mental illnesses, including anxiety, depression, substance use, post-traumatic stress disorder, and relationship challenges. This book empowers clinicians to fit psychotherapy techniques into their preferred appointment lengths. These techniques can be easily used in clinical settings with tight time constraints as each takes about five minutes.

Who Can Benefit From This Book?

Health professionals are increasingly seeing patients who could benefit from emotional wellness support. Waitlists for psychologists and counsellors can be long, so other health professionals are called upon to offer these services. Fortunately, there are a wealth of effective mental health tools that can be taught and practiced in a time-effective manner. The techniques in this book are applicable to many different clinical presentations. For example, Chapter 8 describes how clinicians can use these techniques to more effectively work with patients where there are relationship challenges, including patients with personality disorders. Chapter 10 demonstrates their application in groups ranging from school-aged children to seniors with mild dementia. The techniques can also be used to support caregivers. Lastly, clinicians can use these techniques on themselves to improve wellbeing, prevent burnout, and reach peak flow. In a fast-paced world with high levels of stress, decreased family and social connections, and challenges with work-life balance, everyone can benefit from access to easy-to-use tools for grounding, self-regulation, and increased presence.

Why and When?

The divide between mind and body is arbitrary. Sometimes mental distress manifests as physical symptoms and pain. Physical pain and medical conditions affect mental health. Sometimes trying to address physical complaints without addressing the mental health component leads to multiple "not yet diagnosed" medical conditions and poor response to medication or polypharmacy. Wellness is not just the absence of disease.

Mental health disorders don't just affect the people who suffer from them. They also affect the people around them. Trauma can be transmitted to the next generation. By treating one person, multiple lives can be impacted.

Clinicians only need to find five minutes a day to learn a new strategy and apply it in their practice.

How to Use This Book?

What is helpful for one person will not necessarily be helpful for someone else, so instead of a scripted manual, the first seven chapters teach evidence-based strategies from numerous different schools of psychotherapy.

Each technique has a description, a rationale, and a script to provide the clinician with a ready-to-use presentation of the technique. Some techniques also include additional notes, caveats, sample patient responses, and variations that provide adjustments or alternatives to the original script that might better fit a particular patient.

Practising the technique together with the patient can help to promote connection and healing in the therapeutic relationship.

The rationale of each exercise may be shared with the patient to help them understand why the exercises are important.

The Stage 1 Skills focus on strategies to help the patients:
- Live in the present.
- Be aware of their experience, including their internal world and their body.
- Tolerate their emotions and experience.
- Find language to communicate their experience.
- Allow more positive experiences in their life, to build competence, and be successful.
- Be compassionate towards themselves.
- Develop cognitive flexibility.
- Be effective in their relationships.

The Stage 2 Skills expand on the Stage 1 Skills and are more trauma-specific. However, the Stage 2 Skills may be triggering to some patients. Therefore, it is important for patients to have mastery over some of the Stage 1 Skills, so that they can regulate their emotions using those techniques if they are triggered. Chapter 9 discusses psychological trauma and explains when Stage 2 Skills would be helpful. The later chapters build on the prior ones, so it is recommended to read the whole book in sequential order before applying the Stage 2 Skills. The reader may choose to skip Stage 2 Skills and come back later.

Chapters 8, 9, and 10 describe how the techniques can be applied and how to structure therapy. Chapters 8 and 9 include knowledge sections to provide additional information. Chapter 10 has examples of clinical cases, questions based on the cases, and discussion of potential solutions to help the patient.

Part I: Techniques

CHAPTER 1:
Mindfulness and Body Techniques

Mindfulness has been practiced for thousands of years as an integral part of traditions such as Yoga and Buddhism. Mindfulness techniques are useful to teach the patient early on, because they can help the patient pay attention, be present, and feel calm and grounded, which allows them to work better during psychotherapy. They can be used to treat mood disorders, post-traumatic stress disorder (PTSD), borderline personality disorder (BPD), obsessive-compulsive disorder (OCD), attention deficit hyperactivity disorder (ADHD), addiction / substance abuse, dissociation, and physical symptoms such as chronic pain and somatization disorder.

In the 1900s, Dr. Wilhelm Reich developed the concept of "vegetotherapy," which targeted physical manifestations of emotions to promote healing. In the 1970s, Somatic experiencing was developed by Dr. Peter Levine for treating trauma. Given the connection between the mind and the body, it is important to work with both to improve health.

Mind-Body Connection

Description: Explain to the patients how the mind and the body are connected.

Rationale: Help the patients understand how the techniques in this chapter may help them.

Script: The mind affects the body and the body affects the mind. Your thoughts and mood affect your health. Your health problems affect your mood. By working with the body, you can change how you feel. By working with your mind, you can change how your body feels.

Stage 1 Skills

TECHNIQUE #1: Slow Outbreath

Description: Bring mindfulness to the breath by making the outbreath longer than the inbreath. Use the breath to calm down and bring awareness to the present.

Rationale: The outbreath has a calming effect because it activates the parasympathetic system. The breath is always there and can act as a natural point of focus. It changes with mood and activity. The breath is rhythmic, which is calming. (The same rationale applies to the variations.)

Script: Focus on your breathing. Make your outbreath longer than your inbreath. Notice the coolness of the inbreath and the warmness of the outbreath. Follow the path of your breath from the tip of your nose to your abdomen. Notice the movement of your abdomen. Notice the rhythm of your breathing. If your mind begins to wander, just bring it back to the breath.

Variation A: Progressively Longer Outbreath

Description: Progressively make the outbreath longer.

Script: Make each outbreath slightly longer than the last one. With each outbreath, increase your relaxation.

Variation B: Paced Breathing

Description: Do four counts for the breath in, and six counts for the breath out.

Script: I would like you to breathe in for four counts and breathe out for six counts. Let's practice together, and I will do the counting. One, two, three, four (patient breathes in). One, two, three, four, five, six (patient breathes out). Good. Let's try that a few more times. When you practice at home, I want you to count silently in your mind.

Variation C: Prolonged Outbreath

Description: Focus on prolonging the outbreath for twenty breaths.

Script: I would like you to focus on the breath and make sure that the outbreath is longer than the inbreath. Let's practice for twenty breaths. I'll count each breath from one to twenty. One (patient breathes in and out), two (patient breathes in and out), three (continue counting) ... and finally, twenty.

Variation D: Noticing the Breath at the Tip of the Nose

Description: For those who get uncomfortable during abdominal breathing, remove the script "Notice the movement of your abdomen," and replace it with the following:

Script: Notice the flow in and out of your breath at the tip of your nose.

TECHNIQUE #2: Orienting to the Present

Description: Bring the patient back to the present moment.

Rationale: Even when the danger has passed, sometimes the patient is still stuck in anxiety. Reorienting the patient to the present can help them recognize that the danger has indeed passed. This can help a traumatized patient get out of a flashback. Sometimes focusing on the past brings up regrets and ruminations. Focusing on the uncertainty of the future can bring up anxieties. Staying in the present helps the patient calm down, concentrate, and be thoughtful and mindful about the task at hand. It can help the patient appreciate the present and bring awareness to what they are experiencing: personally, with others, and with their environment.

Script: On a scale of one to ten, ten being fully present, how present are you? What can you do to bring yourself fully to the present? Where does your mind tend to want to go? The past? The future? Whenever you notice your mind wandering, simply bring it back.

TECHNIQUE #3: Engaging the Five Senses

Description: Use the five senses to explore the present.

Rationale: This exercise can help bring the patient to the present.

Script: Using your five senses to notice things around you is very helpful in bringing you back to the present. Tell me five things you see. (Wait for the patient's response. The patient may need prompting e.g., what about this corner of the room?)

Now, tell me:

- Four things you hear (e.g., prompt: What do you hear outside this room?)
- Three things you feel (e.g., prompt: What are you sitting on?)
- Two things you smell (e.g., prompt: Try smelling your hands.)
- One thing you taste (e.g., prompt: What did you last eat?)

Sample response: I see a computer, a phone, a picture, a chair, my hands. I hear the traffic outside, other people talking outside the room, the noise of the fan, myself talking. I feel the chair I'm sitting in, my leg, the clothes on my body. I smell hand sanitizer and cheese from my lunch. I taste cheese from my lunch.

Variation A: Exploring an Object with Five Senses

Description: Exploring an object with five senses.

Rationale: Some patients find it uncomfortable to focus inward on their bodily sensations. Usually these people are able to use their five senses to explore an external object.

Script: Explore this object (e.g., singing bowl) with your five senses.

Sample response: It's brown and gold in colour. It is round. It makes a medium-pitched, sustained ringing sound when struck.

The sound gets slightly louder then slowly dies down. The bowl feels cold, hard, smooth, and heavy. It smells like incense and metal.

Variation B: Use Strong Sensory Input

Description: Use a strong sensory input to bring the patient back to present.

Rationale: This can help bring a patient out of a flashback or dissociative state.

Script: To bring yourself back to the present, you can use something with a strong sensory input, such as the taste of an orange, the smell of lavender, or the taste of toothpaste. Use a stimulus that is not triggering or upsetting.

TECHNIQUE #4: One Mindful Thing

Description: Do one thing at a time mindfully and do not multitask. Practice being in the present moment with one mindful thing.

Rationale: Being mindful is the opposite of being on autopilot. Autopilot mode is frequently used in doing routine tasks and especially while multitasking. It helps conserve cognitive energy but is not very flexible and can lead to errors.

Note: Practice Mindfulness and Engaging the Five Senses using a pleasant or neutral experience first, as a painful experience makes someone want to escape from it and not be present in it. Usually a meal is a positive experience.

Script: I would like you to practice at least once a day using Engaging the Five Senses and One Mindful Thing when you're doing something that you usually do automatically without thinking. This can be when you're walking, standing, sitting, or lying. It can also be used when engaged in tasks like eating, dressing, or waiting. For example, with your next meal, use Engaging the Five Senses and be mindful. Really pay attention to the way your food looks, how it feels as you touch it, and the sensations in your mouth. The sound it makes as you eat it. The smell and taste.

TECHNIQUE #5: Exercise

Description: Do intense exercise when feeling upset or distressed.

Rationale: Exercise releases endorphins and can help with relaxation. Doing intense exercise when upset can help the patient tolerate the distress. It is one way to redirect the negative energy and give the patient a positive reason for feeling shortness of breath and heart palpitations. Trauma involves not being able to move, so exercise and movement can help reduce symptoms related to trauma.

Script: When you're feeling distressed, try exercising intensely. For example, start doing jumping jacks. Notice how you feel.

Variation A: Exercise Regularly

Description: Exercise routinely.

Rationale: Regular exercise can help with mood, sleep, motivation, physical health, etc.

Note: For patients with impaired mobility, adjust to their circumstances and incrementally build on what they are able to do. The therapist may need to work with a physiotherapist, e.g., if a patient is lying in bed, get them to sit up in bed. If they can sit up in bed, see if they can transfer to the chair for meals. Then see if they can transfer to a wheelchair and mobilize out of the room.

Script: The current health recommendation is thirty minutes of exercise a day. I want you to start by doing at least five minutes of regular physical activity daily. If there are certain days of the week that work better for your schedule, you can also do at least ten minutes of exercise three days a week.

TECHNIQUE #6: Mindful Movements

Description: Perform guided mindful movement exercises.

Rationale: Helps calm the patient and bring the patient back to the present moment.

Script: Exercise 1: When you feel ready, get into a comfortable position. Make any adjustments to help yourself feel even more comfortable. Be aware of the way you're moving to help yourself be more comfortable. Do what feels right to you, and feel free to change your position at any point. You're in control.

Exercise 2: Start with standing. Notice your arms by your side and the ground under your feet. Bend your knees slightly to bring even more awareness to your legs and feet. When you're ready, notice the weight shift onto one leg. Notice how your calves feel as you lift the heel of the other foot. Slowly lift the foot and mindfully move forward. Notice how your leg feels through the air. Notice the foot making contact with the floor and how you transfer your weight back to the other foot.

If it feels right to you, try walking slower than usual.

TECHNIQUE #7: Progressive Muscle Relaxation

Description: Progressively tighten and loosen the different muscle groups in your body.

Rationale: Helps the patient notice the difference between tight and relaxed muscles in the different muscle groups. Aids in relaxing muscles.

Note: Before the exercise, remove chewing gum. The patient can skip the eye closing step if they have contact lenses in.

Script: Tense the following muscle groups when you breathe in. Tense them for four to ten seconds, but not to the point of pain or cramping. Suddenly and totally relax that muscle group when you breathe out. Relax for ten to twenty seconds, then move to the next group.

Wrinkle your forehead and make a deep frown.

Close your eyes as tightly as you can.

Clench your jaws and press your lips tightly together.

Make a wide smile.

Shrug your shoulders and raise them toward your ears.

Bend your arms at the elbows and clench your hands into fists.

Bend your hands back at the wrist.

Press the back of your head against the floor or chair.

Touch your chin to your chest. (Try not to create tension in your neck and head.)

Breathe in and hold the breath for four to ten seconds.

Arch your back up and away from the floor or chair.

Engage your stomach.

Squeeze your buttocks tightly together.

Tighten your thighs and calves.

Flex your toes toward your face.

Point your toes away and curl your toes downward.

In a moment, I'm going to count backwards from five to one. When I reach the count of one, you'll be fully back to the present. Five ... four ... three ... two ... one. Now bring yourself back to the present, feeling fully awake, alert, and feeling great.

Variation A: Relax Muscles

Description: Relax the different muscle groups.

Rationale: Helpful for patients who have physical limitations and cannot do certain movements.

Script: Take a deep breath in, and breathe out now. Use the outbreath to help you relax.

Relax the muscles in your face. Relax your scalp, your forehead, your eyebrows, your eyelids, your cheeks, your nose, your mouth, and your lips. Relax your chin and jaw. Make sure your teeth are unclenched. Allow the muscles in your face to relax completely.

Relax your neck. Relax the front part of your neck. Relax the back part of your neck.

Relax your shoulders. Allow your shoulders to relax completely.

Bring your attention back to your breath. Notice the rhythm of your breathing. Notice the movement of your chest. Allow your chest muscles to relax completely.

Relax your stomach muscles. Let go of any tension in that area.

Relax your back muscles. Relax your upper back. Relax your mid back. Relax your lower back. Allow your entire back to relax completely.

Relax your pelvis. Relax your hips. Relax your thighs, your legs, your knees, your calves, your ankles, your feet, and your toes. Let go of any tension in your body. Become completely relaxed.

In a moment, I'm going to count backwards from five to one. When I reach the count of one, you'll be fully back to the present. Five ... four ... three ... two ... one. Now bring yourself back to the present, feeling fully awake, alert, and feeling great.

TECHNIQUE #8: Tapping / Emotional Freedom Technique

Description: Tap various areas of the body and bring mindfulness to them.

Rationale: This is a technique based on acupressure and is used to bring calmness. Rhythms are calming.

Note: The therapist guides the patient through the exercise.

Script: Tap in a rhythmic way at a pressure and speed that makes sense to you. Bring mindful awareness to this. Notice what is happening in your body and mind as you're tapping. Notice your thoughts as you do this. If you find tapping difficult, you can also maintain sustained pressure on the spot.

Tap on the pinky side of your hand.

Tap between your fourth and fifth bone at the back of the hand.

Notice what happens to you when you do this.

Tap above your eyebrows.

Tap over your cheek bones.

Tap below your eyes.

Tap the spot above your upper lip.

Tap on your chin.

Tap on the sensitive spot on your chest that is located one inch below your collarbone and one inch to the sides of your sternum, your breastbone.

Tap between your bottom two ribs.

Notice how you're feeling and what's going on in your body and mind. You may feel more calm or more energized.

TECHNIQUE #9: Diver's Reflex

Description: Hold the breath and put the face in cold water for a few seconds to activate the diver's reflex.

Rationale: Diver's reflex is an innate physiological reaction that occurs in human beings in response to water submersion. When human beings hold their breath in water and the face and nose become wet, physiological changes occur to slow the heart rate and breathing and increase peripheral vascular resistance. The physiological change conserves oxygen and decreases the work of the heart. These changes help the patient feel calm.

Script: When you are feeling distressed, get a bucket of ice water or fill your sink with cold water. Hold your breath and put your face into the cold water. Notice how you feel.

Variation A: Use Ice

Description: Use ice to calm the patient down.

Rationale: Some people might find it difficult to get a bucket of water or fill the sink with ice.

Script: When you are feeling distressed, put ice over your face and nose.

TECHNIQUE #10: Balancing on Uneven Ground

Description: Think while doing a balance exercise.

Rationale: When the balancing system (cerebellar vestibular system) is engaged, it also activates the dorsolateral prefrontal cortex. This is the part of the brain that allows patients to see themselves over time and talk about yesterday and tomorrow, rather than simply live in the moment. It allows them to think about what is happening next and what has happened before.

Note: This can be done on a balance board, trampoline, or BOSU, or just by standing on one foot.

Script: Stand on one foot. I want you to think and stay balanced at the same time. Reflect on your day today. Notice how your thinking changes when you think and balance at the same time.

TECHNIQUE #11: Dual Awareness with Hands

Description: Bring mindful awareness to the hands and the body.

Rationale: Help patients feel safe and feel present in their body.

Note: Some people, especially those who have been traumatized, find it difficult or even terrifying to feel their hand on their chest.

If this occurs, try the exercise on a less threatening part of the body; see the "If not…" script below.

Script: Place your hand on your chest. Notice the spot you're touching underneath your hand. Notice the hand that's touching you. Can you feel the gentleness of your own touch? Notice your chest moving up and down. Can you feel the loving person you're touching? Can you be the hand touching the body and the body being touched by the hand? Can you be and feel both at the same time?

If yes, place the other hand on the abdomen. Can you be and feel both at the same time with this other hand? Now, can you be and feel all four at the same time?

If not and you are unable to feel your hand or the body, try placing your hand in a different location. You can try the back of the other hand, forearm, or arms until you are able to feel the hand. Once you're able to feel your hand, move your hand towards the trunk and try to feel it again. (Repeat the exercise if the patient is able to tolerate it.)

TECHNIQUE #12: Observing Without Words

Description: Practice observing without using words.

Rationale: It helps the patient to be in the moment and to let thoughts go.

Note: Show the patient a photo or painting or image for three minutes. Set a timer.

Script: I want you to observe this image for three minutes without using words in your mind. Try your best to not use words. Observe the thoughts that come into your mind and let them go.

How was the experience for you? What did you notice?

Sample response: The patient might say, "I noticed that it is very challenging not to use words. Words describing the picture keep coming into my head. I find it difficult to focus on the image for three minutes and my mind keeps wandering."

The therapist can validate the experience. "It is challenging to focus on an image for three minutes. It takes practice. Thoughts and words are products of the mind. Good for you for noticing and not judging those thoughts."

TECHNIQUE #13: Mindful Check-in

Description: Have the patient practice regular check-ins with themselves to see if they are still present. Being in autopilot mode is the opposite of being present.

Rationale: Help the patient be aware of whether or not they are in the moment, and bring their awareness back to the present.

Note: Pick an activity where the check-ins would not be dangerous. Some patients may find them distracting. Find a twenty minute period to do frequent check-ins during this technique.

Script: Pick an activity that you usually do automatically and check in with yourself at least ten times during the activity. Notice whether you are present or in autopilot mode. Bring your awareness back to the present and the activity at hand.

What strategies did you find helpful to keep you engaged and present during the activity?

Sample response: I find it easier to stay present when I break tasks up into smaller chunks and mentally say what I'm doing as I'm doing it to keep my mind focused on the task.

TECHNIQUE #14: Changing Body Position to Change Sensation

Description: Change body position and posture to change sensation and feeling.

Rationale: Use the mind-body connection principle to change the sensation or feeling.

Script: 1) Make the body posture for happiness: raise your arms up and smile big. Now try to feel sad. You'll notice that you cannot—your body will not let you feel sad.

Notice how, by changing your posture, you can change the way you feel.

2) Find the posture for anger: e.g., tension in the jaw and fists. Now try tensing and relaxing those muscles.

3) Find the posture for shame: e.g., hunched over, looking down. Move to a more open posture, sit up staring and look up. Move between the posture for shame and the open posture. Go back and forth to reduce the shame. Practice this.

Think of a situation where you felt shame. Notice your posture. Now sit upright with your shoulders back and chin up.

Note: Some people may feel anger. Shame hides and attacks; it protects the self. (See Chapter 7 for strategies on working with shame.)

Stage 2 Skills

Note: Please see the Prologue and Chapter 9 for an explanation of Stage 1 and 2 Skills.

TECHNIQUE #14: Variation A: Exaggerating Body Posture to Heighten Sensation

Description: Exaggerate the body posture to create a stronger sensation.

Rationale: To increase awareness.

Note: This may worsen symptoms, so don't do this variation if the patient is dysregulated.

Script: I notice that you have your fists clenched. I want you to clench them tighter. What happens when you do that? What memories, thoughts, feelings come to mind when you do that? (See Chapter 2 Technique #1: Teaching Language for Emotions and Chapter 5 on working with cognitive distortions / hot thoughts.)

TECHNIQUE #15: Mindfulness about Absentmindedness

Description: The patient keeps track of when they have been absentminded.

Rationale: To bring awareness when times of absentmindedness occur. This can help reduce their recurrence and also help to problem-solve around them.

Note: This exercise may be frustrating. Therefore, the therapist might want to do this with One Mindful Thing or another mindful practice, so the patient can track both absentmindedness and when they were successfully mindful.

Script: What was happening? What were you trying to do? What did you forget to do? What were the consequences?

Sample response: The patient left house keys at work. He was leaving and kept thinking about other things that he still needed to do for work and got distracted. The consequence was that he had to make an extra trip back to the office to get his keys.

TECHNIQUE #16: Mindfulness about Autopilot Mode

Description: Sometimes people go into autopilot mode for routine tasks (e.g., driving). However, errors can occur while someone is in autopilot mode. Building on Technique #15.

Rationale: Reduce errors by helping the patient be aware of autopilot mode.

Script: When the mistake happened, were you on autopilot?

Sample response: I was with my daughter and she handed me a cup. I automatically started to drink from it, and only stopped when she screamed and pulled at my arm. I suddenly realized there was a frog in the cup and she was showing me a frog that she had caught.

TECHNIQUE #17: Mindfulness about Being Present and Being Absentminded

Description: Combine Technique #15 with keeping track of when the patient has been present.

Rationale: The ability to pay attention to awareness is helpful for developing skills to control awareness.

Script: I want you to record daily when you have been absentminded as well as when you have been present. Which Stage 1 Skills did you use to bring yourself back to the present moment when you noticed that you were being absent minded?

TECHNIQUE #18: Mindful Action with Traumatic Memory

Description: Mindfully make an action while thinking of a traumatic memory.

Rationale: Trauma makes people feel helpless and unable to move. Help the patient make the action and move beyond this. They need to realize that the trauma is over and this time it is different. Think and feel while making the action. Mindful awareness helps integration. Help people learn to move to get what they need.

Note: Some patients might find it difficult to hear the word "trauma." They might still be in denial or want to downplay the impact. Other patients find it validating to use the word trauma. The word "difficult" may be substituted for "traumatic" memories.

The therapist needs to adjust the language to what works for their patients.

Script: When thinking of a traumatic memory, is there any action you want to take (that you may have been unable to take previously)?

What are you feeling as you are making this action?

Mindfully take the action you feel you want to take.

Sample response: Patient pushes away with their hands. (The patient was not able to say no and push the perpetrator away during the original traumatic event. In therapy, the patient can now carry out the action mindfully.)

Summary

Given the mind-body connection, changing one changes the other. Working on breathing is a great starting point to calm the mind and body. Mindfulness strategies bring the patient to the present and ground them. These include, engaging the five senses, doing one thing at a time, observing without words, and doing check-ins to get out of autopilot mode.

Ways to work with the body include mindful movement, progressive muscle relaxation, tapping, and dual awareness of using hands to feel the body. Activating the diver's reflex with ice helps with relaxation, and initiating the balance system is anti-dissociating. Stage 2 Skills may worsen the patient's symptoms, so practice emotional regulation Stage 1 Skills until the patient feels ready to progress. By exaggerating body posture to heighten sensation and using mindful action, the patient can process the traumatic memory. Being mindful of mistakes that occurred while the patient was absentminded, being aware of autopilot mode, and focusing on being present versus absentminded help the patient to stay in the moment.

CHAPTER 2:
Metacognition / Mentalizing

In the 1990s, Mentalization-Based Therapy was first developed by Dr. Peter Fonagy and Dr. Anthony Bateman to treat borderline personality disorder. Metacognition, or the ability to mentalize, is a more advanced level of reasoning where you think about thinking.

Metacognitive skills usually develop from parents being attuned to their child. Parents wonder about a child's state of mind, explore what the child thinks and feels, and what motivates them. However, some patients did not have attuned parents who helped them develop these skills. In this case, the therapist can help patients develop metacognitive skills by creating a safe space and encouraging self-reflection and self-exploration. The patient can think about state of mind, emotions, knowledge, behaviour, self, and other people. This chapter covers the first five. Thinking about others is covered in Chapter 6 Interpersonal Therapy (IPT).

State of Mind: You can bring awareness to your state of mind by identifying it and monitoring its accuracy. You may begin by noticing how organized or disorganized your state of mind is.

Emotion: Metacognition on emotions enhances your ability to identify your mood and its intensity. Think about what's making you feel this way.

Knowledge: You may be able to see beyond the information that's given to you. You appreciate the limitations of knowledge and are sensitive to the context and the underlying assumptions.

Behaviour: Having an awareness of your action plans helps keep you proactive. Think about prior actions and their context. You consider and optimize the options.

Self: Metacognition on the self means thinking about the concept of "self" and its meaning.

Other people: You can take on the perspective of other people and appreciate that different people can have different opinions about the same event. You are aware of the interconnection and interdependence between people. You develop compassion and empathy for others. You understand more complex relationships and systems.

State of Mind

1) Automatic thinking versus slow, controlled thinking.

2) Thinking about self versus others.

3) Thinking about what's going on within (internal) versus focusing on the outside world (external).

4) Thinking versus feeling (the "wise mind" in dialectical behaviour therapy is when someone can think and feel simultaneously).

5) Focusing on the past versus present.

Splitting occurs when someone is at an extreme and can only see one or the other state of mind but not both. It is important to work on being able to simultaneously balance the opposite states. (See Chapter 5 Technique #1: Cognitive Distortions / Hot Thoughts for All or Nothing Thinking.)

Stage 1 Skills

TECHNIQUE #1: Teaching Language for Emotions

Description: Develop a language for emotions such as anger, sadness, happiness, fear, curiosity, surprise, disgust, love, guilt, and shame.

Rationale: Help the patient find language for themselves to be able to communicate emotions. Learning words for their experiences can help those who are psychosomatic to identify the "symptoms" (e.g., heart palpitation) that are associated with an emotional state.

Script: E.g., What is anger? How do you feel in your body when you feel angry?

—Anger is the feeling I get when I feel violated and I want people to back off.

Variation A: Act Out the Emotion

Description: Have a deck of cards with different emotions written on them. The therapist and the patient take turns acting out the emotion and guessing what is being acted out.

Rationale: Help patients identify the emotion of the other person and mindfully act out the emotion.

Script: We are going to take turns drawing cards and acting out the emotion on the card. Whoever isn't drawing the card will guess the emotion.

TECHNIQUE #2: Addressing Fears and Myths about Emotions

Description: Explore the patient's fears about their emotions by discussing them.

Rationale: Emotions give information. Emotions help people plan, act quickly, and connect with others. Some people are afraid of their own emotions.

Script: I am going to read out each statement. Tell me whether you believe this is true or false, or the extent to which you believe this on a scale of one to ten, ten being you fully believe this.

Each of the following is a myth about emotions. This means they are untrue statements that some people might believe. Let's go through each one and discuss it.

- Feeling emotions is a sign of weakness or it means not being in control.
- There's a correct way to feel.
- Negative emotions are the result of bad attitudes.

- Intense emotions help you achieve your goals.
- You are your emotions.
- It is disingenuous to change your emotions.
- Always trust your emotions.
- People who are free act on their emotions.
- Emotions occur without reason.

TECHNIQUE #3: Window of Tolerance / Identifying the Intensity of Emotions

Description: Dr. Dan Siegel coined the phrase "window of tolerance." The window of tolerance is the optimal level of emotional intensity that allows the patient to think and feel at the same time.

Rationale: Discuss the window of tolerance to help patients be aware of and stay in their window of tolerance.

The purpose is not to control emotions but rather to tolerate them. Think of emotions as waves. Learn to surf your emotions.

In the hyperarousal state, the patient is experiencing intense emotions and is unable to think. The patient may be using addiction to cope with the intense emotion. (See Chapter 9 Knowledge #10: Pathological Self-soothing / Addiction.)

In the hypoarousal state, the patient is shut down and may be dissociated or numb. The patient may be unable to feel emotions.

Sometimes patients oscillate between hyperarousal and hypoarousal. The therapist helps the patient regulate their emotion (see Chapter 1 Stage 1 Skills.)

Note: Some therapists use the term "Subjective Units of Distress" (SUDS) and ask the patient on a scale of zero to a hundred how distressed they are.

Script: Identify the intensity of the emotion on a scale of zero to a hundred (or zero to ten.)

At what level of arousal do you function the most optimally? What skills can you use to help you get to that level of arousal and stay within your window of tolerance?

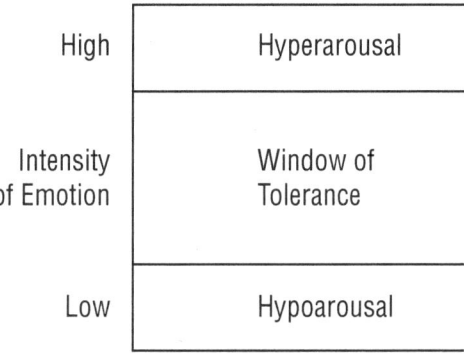

Figure 1: Window of Tolerance

TECHNIQUE #4: Judgments Versus Facts

Description: Think about knowledge and distinguish between judgments and facts.

Rationale: Judgments sometimes act like oil on a fire; they can intensify negative emotions. Patients' negative criticisms of themselves are what cause suffering.

Script: Facts are things you can prove. Judgments are opinions.

Notice judgments, but don't judge them. Think of thoughts as products of your mind. Just because you thought it doesn't mean it's true or real.

Observe the thought without judgment. Don't deny it or suppress it. Don't cling to it. Don't try to make it larger or smaller. Allow thoughts to come and go. Simply be open and aware. Think of the facts of who, what, when, and where, without the judgment.

TECHNIQUE #5: Creating Distance with Mentalizing

Description: Create cognitive distance by mentalizing and speaking *for* a part rather than *from* the part.

Rationale: Mentalizing creates distance from emotion and helps the patient think and feel at the same time.

Script: You cannot control events, but you can influence your reaction to the event.

You construct your experiences and learn from them. You are not your experiences.

Your sensory input plus mind processing are the construct of the experience. Experience changes. Each person has their own subjectively constructed reality.

Imagine that you are speaking for the angry or hurt part rather than from the angry or hurt part.

E.g., "I hate you." (Speaking from the angry part.)

"I feel angry when…" (Speaking for the part.)

TECHNIQUE #6: Identifying States of Mind, Balanced Perspectives

Description: Help the patient identify the different states of mind and which one they are in.

Rationale: This can help them balance their perspective.

Script: Which state of mind are you in?

E.g., Patient talking about an emotionally upsetting experience but there's a lack of affect. (Focus on cognition.)

Therapist says, "How does that make you feel?" (Shifting focus from cognition to feeling.)

E.g., Patient talks about how she feels.

"What thoughts were going through your mind when you were feeling this way?"

E.g., Patient talks about herself the whole time. (Focus on self and what's going on within self.)

Therapist validates the patient's feelings and then asks the patient, "What do you think the other person was thinking or feeling?" (Shifting focus from self to others.)

"What was going on in the environment at that time?" (Shifting focus from internal to external.)

Balance the perspective.

E.g., Help the patient think and feel at the same time. "How does that make you feel? What are your thoughts?"

TECHNIQUE #7: Using Scale for Awareness

Description: States of mind on a scale.

Rationale: Use a scale to help patients bring awareness. By bringing awareness to how organized their mind is during therapy, the patient can become more organized.

Script: On a scale of zero to ten:

How organized or disorganized is your state of mind? How do you know if you're disorganized (e.g., lack of flow, changing state, mind scattered, etc.)?

How much are you focused on the past versus focused on the present? (Patient learns to focus on the present.)

How much are you focused on yourself versus others?

Bringing awareness to signs of change.

On a scale of zero to ten, where are you at? If you're at eight now, how would you know if you have moved to a seven?

TECHNIQUE #8: Therapist Attunement for Awareness

Description: Therapist being attuned to the patient and pointing things out.

Rationale: Sometimes patients have difficulty being attuned to themselves. The therapist helps point things out to bring awareness.

Script: I notice the movement in your body.

E.g., I noticed you are clenching your fist. How are you feeling? You seem frustrated.

What do you feel compelled to do?

E.g., I feel compelled to punch the wall.

When patient is disorganized:

"Let's slow down. You're disorganized." (Therapist gives patient feedback during the clinic to foster awareness.)

Variation A: Therapist Demonstrating Metacognitive Skills

Description: The therapist mentalizes their own experience in a curious and nonjudgmental way. What's going on with me? The therapist communicates openly and genuinely.

Rationale: The therapist teaches the patient about attunement by demonstrating it.

Script: "I feel uncomfortable when you do…"

"That sounds like a really intense story. I feel angry when I hear this story. Let's take a moment to work on regulating together." (See Chapter 1 Stage 1 Skills.)

TECHNIQUE #9: Reflecting on Behaviour

Description: Explore and help patients reflect on their own behaviour.

Rationale: Once you understand where the patient is coming from, then you can reframe this as it served a function previously. (See reframing in Chapter 3.)

Script: What compels you to do this (behaviour)? What does this (behaviour) do for you? How does this protect you? How did it serve you in the past? How did it help you survive? What are you afraid might happen if you let go of this emotion e.g., shame? What are the pros and cons of this (behaviour)?

Sample response: I stayed in bed all day. When my parents were fighting, I stayed out of their way. It helped me to save energy. Why bother when it wouldn't change anything? It helped me survive, because I wouldn't get caught up in the fighting. If I start doing things, then people will have expectations of me. I'm afraid of disappointing others. I'm afraid of losing disability funding. The pros of this behaviour are that people don't expect much of me, so I don't have to worry about disappointing others or losing disability funding. The cons are that I feel bad about myself, not being able to contribute much. I might feel better if I started doing things.

TECHNIQUE #10: Curiosity and "I Wonder" Statements

Description: Using curiosity to help the patient explore within themselves.

Rationale: Helps the patient be curious about themselves to reflect and understand themselves better.

Script: I'm curious about how ___ (e.g., your anger) has helped you.

Sample response: My anger pushed people away and that helped me feel safe. Anger also keeps me motivated.

Can you explain that? Tell me more.

What makes you believe that?

Where do those thoughts and feelings come from?

How long have you felt this way? When did you first have these feelings?

Variation A: "I Wonder" Statement

Description: Help patients reflect with "I wonder" statements.

Rationale: "I wonder" statements also bring curiosity.

Script: I wonder what would be useful for you.

I wonder if this has brought up some sensitivities. (Sometimes patients use anger to push the therapist away and avoid sensitive topics.)

TECHNIQUE #11: Pros and Cons

Description: Create a pros and cons list.

Rationale: Helps the patient explore both sides.

Script: E.g., What are the pros and cons of getting better?

What are the pros and cons of staying sick?

Variation A: Explore Pros and Cons by Using a Story

Description: For those who have difficulty thinking of themselves, use a story.

Rationale: Some patients may be too dysregulated when they start thinking of themselves. Using a story can help provide some distance from the intense emotions and still allow them to explore both sides.

Script: Mr. A lost both arms in an accident. He gets financial support from the government, support from his family, as well as a personal support worker. Now there's new technology that will allow him to have a new set of arms. What are the pros and cons of getting this new set of arms?

TECHNIQUE #12: Journaling

Description: Encourage the patient to journal for themselves.

Rationale: Journaling encourages a deep self-reveal and fosters awareness.

Note: The patient doesn't need to share the content with the therapist, but the therapist is open to hearing about it if the patient chooses to share.

Script: Write about triggers and what leads to the emotion. The level of intensity. How they felt, thought, and behaved. Write about sources of stress which can be health, family, friends, work, etc.

Stage 2 Skills

TECHNIQUE #13: Observing Emotions

Description: Observe emotions without judging, magnifying, or shrinking them.

Rationale: Natural emotions come and go quickly when the patient doesn't fuel them with judgment. Observe them without running away or distracting yourself.

Script: Notice the feeling of sadness. Notice the intensity of it and observe how it comes and naturally ends. No emotions last forever. Let emotions run their course.

TECHNIQUE #14: Bringing Awareness to Self

Description: Bring awareness to the self and combine skills from Chapters 1 and 2.

Rationale: Practicing observation and letting go of judgments allows people to let things be, rather than try to control them. It helps the patient change from "doing" mode (especially autopilot mode) to "being" mode. This helps with building tolerance of their emotions and experiences. Observing helps people notice that things are always changing and no moment lasts forever. Terrible things will end and suffering is not forever.

Note: Some people may find this triggering. If this occurs, remind them about being nonjudgmental.

Script: Bring awareness to yourself. Reconnect with yourself. Be mindful.

What is going on inside of you? Observe your emotions, thoughts, and behaviour. Be curious and nonjudgmental about what you notice.

How are you feeling?

Where in your body do you feel this? (Activate an interoceptive pathway to bring calm and agency.)

What happened that made you feel this way? How are you reacting to it?

What thoughts are associated with this?

What do you do and how do you behave when you feel this way? What do you need to do?

What are the outcomes of feeling this emotion?

What does this say about you?

Variation A: Using the Body Scan for Interoception

Script: 1) Body Scan:

    a) Notice the sensations in the body.

    b) Scan your body for areas of tension and release the tension.

    c) Bring awareness to your breath.

2) Notice your feelings and emotions.

3) Notice any thoughts that come up. Observe the experience. If there are any judgments, let them go.

4) Orient to the present: Where are you now? How old are you? How tall are you?

This exercise can be combined with the Chapter 1 Technique #3 exercise. The patient can be asked to bring attention first to the self (with this exercise), then shift the attention to the environment (Chapter 1 Technique #3), and notice that shift in attention.

Summary

Mentalizing is a critical skill that helps patients become aware and reflect on their state of mind, emotions, knowledge, behaviour, self, and other people. This awareness helps patients to balance their perspectives, organize their thoughts, and focus on the present. Exploring pros and cons also helps them balance their perspective. Patients need to be able to identify their emotions, so they can work on staying within their window of tolerance. The ability to distinguish between facts and judgements and to reduce judgments help with emotional regulation. Cognitive distance from negative emotions can be created by mentalizing and speaking for a part rather than from the part. The therapist can help foster mentalizing skills by being attuned to the patient, demonstrating the skills, and helping patients be curious about themselves. Patients can work on self-reflective ability by journaling and nonjudgmentally observing their emotions, thoughts, behaviour, and bodily sensations. Mentalizing and self-reflection create understanding and improve emotional wellbeing.

CHAPTER 3:
Fostering Positive Experiences

In the 1950s, Dr. Abraham Maslow coined the term "positive psychology." Then, Dr. Martin Seligman researched, taught, and published books on positive psychology. In contrast to the medical model that focuses on illnesses, positive psychology focuses on people's strengths and positive experiences.

It is important to foster positive experiences, because the absence of negative beliefs doesn't mean the patient acquires positive beliefs. A person cannot make negative experiences go away, but can balance them with positive experiences making the negative emotions more tolerable. By working on the patient's strengths, they can become more confident and competent.

However, some patients can find positive emotions triggering and need help to increase their tolerance for these feelings. Pleasure may be associated with danger. It may not previously have been safe to express positive feelings, or patients may feel they're not worthy. A pleasurable event may have been followed by a dangerous event causing the pleasurable event to become a trigger. If the patient has difficulty tolerating positive emotions, check-in with the patient and slow down. Engage in positive emotions and take it to the patient's limit of tolerance, then return to regulation, then go back to a positive experience. Build capacity for positive experiences by asking the patient to be present and stay with the positive experience for as long as they are able to tolerate it. Invite the patient to notice the positive feelings in the body as well as the discomfort. Reassure them that over time the discomfort will diminish. People are surrounded by opportunities to notice and to create positive experiences. Help the patient bring awareness to these opportunities.

Stage 1 Skills

TECHNIQUE #1: Self-Care

Description: Take care of yourself. Live well, exercise, have a healthy diet, sleep, get treatment for any illnesses, and establish a routine. This includes emotional, physical, social, and spiritual self-care.

Rationale: Physical health affects mental health. Refer to the mind-body connection in Chapter 1. Self-care is not selfish. People need to take care of themselves before taking care of others.

Script: Do what you need to take care of yourself and live well. Aim to do at least thirty minutes of exercise each day. Eat well: consume more fresh fruits and vegetables, drink water, cut back on juice and pop, fatty food, or junk food. Get enough sleep: on average people need around eight hours of sleep per night. Get treatment for any illnesses. See your doctors. Establish a routine.

Start by doing one of these things and devote at least five minutes a day to self-care.

TECHNIQUE #2: Addressing Vulnerabilities

Description: Address vulnerabilities to increase the window of tolerance.

Rationale: Helps the patients regulate their emotions better.

Script: What makes you vulnerable to being emotionally dysregulated?

E.g., being hungry, needing to use the washroom, not getting enough sleep, working long hours, being in a noisy place, etc.

What can you do to address this?

Try eating regular meals, taking regular breaks, etc.

TECHNIQUE #3: Positive Activities

Description: Engage in positive activities.

Rationale: Helps people figure out what they enjoy, so they start to focus on the positives and balance their perspective (away from focusing on negatives.)

Note: Some people with difficulty navigating interpersonal relationships may find it easier to work with animals.

Script: Do activities that help you connect with others and get back in sync with others. For example:

- Tossing a ball back and forth
- Singing together, chanting or praying together
- Dancing, martial arts, or boxing

Do activities that calm you and bring you pleasure and safety. For example:

- Tai chi, Qigong, yoga, including trauma-informed yoga
- Swings, walks in nature
- Rhythm, music, drumming, clapping
- Hugging a friend, petting a cat
- Weighted blanket, rocking chair

Do activities that allow you to play a different role. For example:

- Acting and drama, including psychodrama

TECHNIQUE #4: Reframing

Description: Seeing things as "glass half full" rather than "glass half empty."

Rationale: Reframing to focus on the positives.

Script: Reframe beliefs about self. For example:

- Rather than saying "I'm bad," reframe it as "Good people can make bad decisions."

Move towards positives, rather than moving away from negatives. What would you rather see, do, feel instead? For example:

- Instead of saying "I don't want to do ___," say "I want to do ___."
- Instead of saying "I hate my job," what would you rather see at your job?
- "I want to stop drinking." What would you be doing if you could stop drinking?
- "I want to stop feeling anxious." How do you want to feel instead?

Changing the wording helps change how people feel. This helps them think of the future from a different point of view.

You can also reframe problematic behaviours that a patient uses to cope or self-soothe (as solutions to a problem), for example, an eating disorder, substance abuse, self-harm, and dissociation. For example:

- Therapist: You were feeling distressed. Cutting yourself released endorphins and helped you feel relaxed. You were trying to cope and self-soothe. Would you like me to show you another technique for self-soothing? It doesn't work as well as cutting, but it also doesn't cause harm.

Saying "Don't do this" may make the patient feel guilt or shame and worsen problematic coping behaviour. The patient may also get upset at the clinician for judging them and might say, "Don't tell me what to do." Instead, reframe. For example:

- Therapist: I see patients with dissociative identity as having multiple talents: a talent for self-hypnosis and a talent for multiple voices. Dissociation helped you cope with unbearable situations and allowed you to keep information from yourself so you could still have a relationship with your caregivers.

People get pathologized. Instead of thinking about a medical diagnosis and labels, try to understand where they're coming from and understand how they see their world.

TECHNIQUE #5: Happiness and Positives

Description: Exploring what brings happiness and positivity.

Rationale: Helps patients figure out what makes them happy.

Note: If a patient has difficulty identifying a time when they were happy or focusing on the positive, try the following variations.

Script: What do you enjoy? What makes you happy?

What in your environment brings you enjoyment? E.g., Animals.

What memories bring you happiness, or when in your life have you felt happy? What was it that gave you that feeling? Who was there and what was around you?

What are the things that went well today, even if they are small? E.g., The things that went well today are: I met up with a friend, and I finished my essay.

What are you grateful for? E.g., I'm grateful for having a place to live. (It may be helpful to write a list of what you are grateful for.)

Who are the people that you feel care about you?

Variation A: Magic Wand

Description: Use imagination to think of what would be different.

Script: If there's a magic wand and you are suddenly much better, what would be different? How will you know when things are improved?

Variation B: Less Bad

Description: Think of what is slightly less than the worst case scenario.

Script: Think of a time when you coped better than your worst moments, or a time when you felt less bad. What's one thing you didn't forget or miss today?

TECHNIQUE #6: Self-Compassion

Description: Be compassionate and kind toward yourself.

Rationale: Patients sometimes have a harsh inner critic. This often is not helpful and brings misery. Self-compassion helps people feel happier, more motivated, and satisfied.

Script: 1) Notice and acknowledge your suffering. Be kind, understanding, and supportive of yourself.

It is understandable that you feel this way. It is important and okay to take the time you need.

Suffering and imperfection are parts of being human.

Treat yourself like you would treat a friend or a loved one.

What would you say to a friend experiencing the same thing?

What would a friend say to you?

2) Wish yourself well.

E.g., May I feel healthy and well. May I feel ___ (give yourself whatever words you need.)

Send those same wishes to others.

Try talking to yourself in a different tone, a kinder tone.

Motivate yourself without using criticism.

E.g., Everyone has something they can improve on.

It takes courage to admit your weaknesses and flaws. They don't define you.

TECHNIQUE #7: Values

Description: Know your values.

Rationale: This is part of getting to know who you are and helps make life meaningful.

Script: What's important to you? What guides you and gives you motivation? List three things that are important to you or guide you and give you motivation.

Examples of values: Accomplishments, career, creativity, fame, family, growth, health, independence, integrity, justice, kindness, knowledge, love, money, peace, power, relationships, respect, safety, spirituality, and truth.

TECHNIQUE #8: Setting Boundaries

Description: Set boundaries with other people and be assertive.

Rationale: Once you know your values, it's easier to set boundaries. For people whose boundaries were violated earlier in life, setting boundaries can be more difficult. Setting boundaries can reveal priorities and protect what's important in one's life.

Script: Make yourself a priority. Set limits and be assertive. Be aware of your thoughts and feelings. Get support.

There wasn't anything you could have done to prevent your abuse in childhood, but now there are things you can do to prevent abuse.

TECHNIQUE #9: Setting Goals

Description: Help your patient set goals and figure out ways to achieve them.

Rationale: Helps the patient build confidence and competence.

Script: 1) Write down your goal. State the goal to yourself or others. What do you want to achieve? What motivates you to do this? Be specific and realistic.

2) Get organized. Have a to-do list on a phone or in a notebook and keep it easily accessible (carry it with you.) You might want to use an alert or alarm function if you're using a to-do list on your phone.

Prioritize: Which task is more important, urgent, or rewarding?

How will you achieve the goal?

Break it down into small, achievable steps. (This is less overwhelming and the patient will do better when they are less stressed.)

3) Set a timeline. Consider long-term and short-term goals.

4) Focus on positives rather than negatives. Think of things you are going to do rather than things you are going to stop doing.

TECHNIQUE #10: Problem Solving

Description: Help patients identify and solve problems.

Rationale: Help patients be self-sufficient and have the skills to navigate through challenges. This builds confidence and fosters a capacity for problem solving.

Script: What frustrates you?

What gets in your way?

What can you do about it?

What's working, or what has worked in the past?

Start by writing down as many solutions as you can without judging them.

What are the pros and cons of the solutions?

What is the best solution?

Once you have made the decision, try to love your decision. What are the consequences of indecision (e.g., not doing a good job on either of the decisions, frustration, self-criticism, and stress)?

If the patient reports drinking as a "social thing," invite them to consider solutions. Holding a non-alcoholic beverage, finding new friends, setting limits, etc.

Variation A: When the Problem is Not Present

Script: When do you not have the problem? How did you manage to keep the problem from worsening?

E.g., You got out of your house today when you previously stayed at home most of the time. How did you manage that? What's working? Tell me more.

TECHNIQUE #11: Mastery and Competence

Description: Steps to take to get better at something.

Help the patient figure out what they are good at. Help them discover what they can do at their capacity. If a patient can't work at a job, they can at least volunteer. If work is not going well, they may need accommodations or reduced hours.

Work on their hobbies and what helps them with happiness, self-esteem, and empowerment. It may be helpful to work with a recreational therapist.

Play to their strengths.

E.g., Patients who are artists may do better with art therapy. People with dissociative disorders tend to be easier to hypnotize and may do well with hypnotherapy.

Rationale: Work can be helpful in building routine, behaviour activation, socializing, building confidence, and finding meaning. Help patients find balance and be successful.

Script: Have you thought about returning to work? Have you discussed returning to work with your employer? What about volunteering? What do you want to do? What do you feel is reasonable for you to handle?

What are your hobbies? What are you willing to try?

TECHNIQUE #12: Self-Esteem

Description: Working on building self-esteem.

Rationale: Some people try to compensate for low self-esteem by doing. These people can temporarily feel good about themselves but they can fall back into feeling "not good enough." Self-esteem is about being and not about doing.

Script: Name things you are proud of.

Think about a time when you felt really good about yourself.

Name your positive qualities and your strengths.

Think of a time when you made an impact.

Think of a time when you were at your best. What did that look like, sound like, feel like?

Think of positive interactions you've had with other people.

Think about feeling good about yourself with other people.

Think about getting the response you want from other people.

Hold on to feeling good about yourself more frequently and for longer periods of time. Journal on how long you can hold on to feeling good about yourself in different situations. Then work on feeling good about yourself in situations that are the most challenging for you. Move from doing to being, so that you can feel good about yourself just by being.

Variation A: Imagining Making an Impact

Description: Alternative to thinking of a time when they have made an impact.

Note: Use the variations if the patient has trouble coming up with examples for the above technique:

Script: Imagine yourself making an impact and what you would want to do in that situation.

Variation B: Count Little Things

Description: Count the little things and what's working.

Script: You asked for help and that takes strength and courage.

TECHNIQUE #13: Fostering Hope and Optimism

Description: Instil hope in the patient.

Rationale: The patient needs hope to be motivated to work towards a better future. Focusing on the positives can bring positive outcomes. This is called a self-fulfilling prophecy; a person's expectation leads them to behave in a way that confirms their belief.

Note: The therapist also needs to have hope for the patient and believe that people can get better. Therapists can try thinking of something they like or admire about their patient to encourage positive feelings towards that patient.

(Also see Techniques #4: Reframing and #9: Setting Goals.)

Script: What's one thing you are looking forward to in the next week? (Future orientation.)

All bad things come to an end. (Remind them that nothing lasts forever, and instil a sense of time.)

What does it mean to live well given your current limitations?

E.g., If a patient is unable to walk due to a spinal cord injury, they can still do upper body exercise and stay fit.

TECHNIQUE #14: Finding Meaning

Description: Help the patient find meaning in their life.

Rationale: Help patients feel there's a purpose and reason to live. Help them feel that they have it within themselves to do something special or meaningful.

Script: What matters the most to you?

What's your favourite part of what you're doing?

What's the most meaningful part of what you're doing?
What made you want to do what you do?
What makes you proud of what you're doing?
How do you know you make a difference?
What makes it a good day?

TECHNIQUE #15: Building Resilience

Description: Resilience is the ability to have favourable outcomes despite adversity.

These habits increase resilience:
- Sense of agency or mastery, skills, independence
- Routines and predictability, safety
- Finding purpose and meaning, giving back, faith
- Supportive relationships (guidance, nurturing, protection), community and social support, sense of belonging
- Health
- Finances, housing
- Positive attitude

Rationale: Strengthen the patient, so they are able to handle adversity.

Script: How did you survive that?

What are you good at? What did you do to find meaning? What are your supports?

What can you do to further strengthen these?

TECHNIQUE #16: Combining Techniques from Chapters 1 and 3

Description: Mindful check-in with the mental and/or physical to-do list. Practice mindfulness and relaxation skills before tackling tasks.

Rationale: Doing complex tasks or having multiple conflicting goals can be stressful. Combine mindfulness strategies to improve success in reaching goals.

Script: Before doing a task, state your goal. Think of what you are doing and why. If the task is complex, break it up into smaller steps and set priorities. Before starting the task, do a mindfulness exercise such as slowing the outbreath. While doing the task, check-in mindfully with yourself by referring to your mental or physical to-do list and make sure you're still on track with your goal.

TECHNIQUE #17: Combining Techniques from Chapters 2 and 3

Description: Pros and cons, awareness, and problem solving.

Rationale: Help patients see both perspectives, understand themselves, and then come up with a solution.

Script: What are the pros and cons of self-harm?

What does it do for you?

How long does the release from self-harm last?

What are alternatives or opposite actions that you can take?

Let's solve this problem together.

Stage 2 Skills

TECHNIQUE #18: Rewriting Your Story and Reframing

Description: Rewrite the story from the perspective of self-compassion.

Rationale: The earlier chapters of the story influence the later chapters, but the later chapters are yet to be written. Help people get unstuck and reframe this in a way that incorporates more positives. Integrate the traumatic experience into their bigger life story. The traumatic experience is part of their identity, but not their whole identity. It can be isolating when someone is not able to convey their inner experience.

Script: What's your story?

Sometimes people get stuck in their story, for example, always perceiving themselves as victims.

You create your narrative.

How do you feel without that story?

You don't need to hang on to the story if it's not serving you well.

You can live your life or you can live your story.

Be curious: What does that story say about you?

What gave you comfort?

Your past is only one part of your story; it is not the whole story.

TECHNIQUE #19: Self-Forgiveness

Description: Forgive yourself.

Rationale: Holding onto self-hatred and loathing is not helpful. Self-forgiveness reduces shame and promotes recovery from setbacks.

Script: You didn't have the information or the insight that you have now.

Who are the people that played a role in this event? How much responsibility did each one of them have with regards to the outcome?

Humans make mistakes.

Everyone indulges and slips up sometimes. Don't be so hard on yourself. Just try again.

TECHNIQUE #20: Forgiving Others

Description: Forgive others.

Rationale: Forgiving can help reduce anger.

Caveat: Forgiveness may be tricky. Forgiveness too early may be invalidating to the patient. Only invite the patient to forgive if it feels right to the patient and they feel ready to do so.

Script: List people you forgive.

I forgive…

Summary

Self-care is important for both physical and mental well-being. Help the patient explore things they like and engage in positive activities so they will feel happy, calm, connected to others. Reframing moves patients towards a more positive frame of mind. Self-compassion and gratitude help people feel happier and more satisfied. When a patient explores their values, they can set healthy boundaries. Through setting and reaching goals, patients can gain a sense of mastery and competence.

Self-esteem is about being and not about doing, so by practicing holding onto good feelings about themselves, patients can improve their self-esteem. It is important to help patients build a healthy sense of self-esteem, so play to the patient's strengths and build resilience. Fostering positive experiences help patients find meaning, have hope and make life worth living.

CHAPTER 4:
Using Imagination / Hypnotic Techniques

In the late 1700s, Dr. Franz Mesmer began investigating the phenomenon of "mesmerism." Dr. James Braid coined the term "hypnotism" in the 1800s. Dr. Milton Erickson founded the American Society for Clinical Hypnosis in the 1900s.

Hypnosis is a method of inducing trances. It can change attention, perceptions, beliefs, emotions, behaviours, and bodily sensations to improve self-esteem, concentration, sports performance, and weight control. Hypnosis can be used to treat mental illnesses, including mood disorders, OCD, sexual problems, insomnia, addiction, PTSD, and dissociation. It can also help ease physical problems, including pain, irritable bowel syndrome (IBS), nausea in pregnancy, and high blood pressure.

Hypnosis was previously the treatment of choice for PTSD. Currently, eye movement desensitization and reprocessing (EMDR) is one of the preferred treatments for simple PTSD. A connection between hypnosis and EMDR is that the eye movement used in EMDR is also noted in patients who are under hypnosis.

One of the key elements of hypnotherapy is using imagination. This chapter covers using imagination and hypnotic techniques. The following hypnotic techniques do not need to be combined with a formal hypnotic induction. Although formal hypnotic inductions are beyond the scope of this book, a strategy for self-hypnosis is covered. Imagination or hypnotic techniques help people open up to new possibilities, habits, and patterns. Hypnosis can be calming. People who are traumatized and dissociating tend to have a natural ability for self-hypnosis. Sometimes traumatized patients can go into trance even without a formal hypnotic induction by simply using the following hypnotic techniques.

These scripts can be added to the following techniques.

For the beginning of the technique: "Either soften your gaze or close your eyes, whichever feels more comfortable to you." (This can help enhance relaxation and imagination.)

For the middle of the technique: See Script for each of the techniques.

For the end of the technique: "I'm going to count backwards from five to one. When I reach the count of one, you will be fully awake, alert, and feeling great. Five ... four ... three ... two ... eyes starting to open, one, eyes wide open, feeling fully awake, alert, settled with the experience, and feeling great."

Stage 1 Skills

TECHNIQUE #1: Imagining a Safe Place

Description: Imagine a safe place. Describe a fantasy place using all five senses. Ask the patient to write their scripts at home and bring them to the clinic.

End with "You are happy, calm, safe, and secure. You are in control."

Rationale: Help the patients find a safe place and calm down.

Sample Script: You are bathing in the warm water of the lagoon. You are sitting on white sand. You lean against smooth black volcanic rocks. You see the light blue water of the lagoon. The water has a faint salty smell and taste to it. You see and feel the ripples in the water. There are houses of various colours in the distance. There's a bright blue, a bright red, and a bright yellow house in the first row. You feel the soft wind blow gently on your body. You hear the rustling of trees in the distance. You hear the soft chirping of birds. You see the blue sky with some soft cotton candy-like clouds slowly drifting by. You feel the warmth of the sun on your skin. You feel the warm water gently soothing your body. You are happy, calm, safe, and secure. You are in control.

TECHNIQUE #2: Imagining a Personal Bubble

Description: Patients imagine a bubble that is under their control.

Rationale: This creates a safe personal space and the patient can regulate the feeling of closeness or distance to the therapist.

Script: Imagine your own personal bubble. It is a perfectly safe environment that only you can access. You can adjust and re-adjust the size of the bubble until it feels just right. It is not too big that you lose the sense of safety from being in a bubble, and not too small that you feel claustrophobic. You can move the bubble around the room to whatever location feels right for you. At any point, you can move the bubble and adjust how close or how far you are from me.

TECHNIQUE #3: Mood Dial

Description: Imagine a dial that controls the intensity of your emotions.

Rationale: A metaphor for the window of tolerance. It may help patients better regulate their emotions. Patients with dissociation may need to dial up the intensity of emotions so they feel something. On the other hand, patients with anxiety may need to dial down the intensity of the emotion.

Script: Imagine a dial, like the heat knob on the stove. Imagine making a stew; if the heat is too high, the stew will boil over or burn. If there's no heat, then nothing is cooking. You want to find the optimal heat for making this stew. Imagine being able to dial up or dial down the intensity of your emotion so that it is at a level which you can tolerate and at a level where you function optimally.

TECHNIQUE #4: Chronic Pain Management Techniques

Description: Techniques for coping with chronic pain.

Rationale: A non-pharmacological method for pain management using the concept of the mind-body connection.

Caveat: Make sure the patient has had a proper medical work-up for pain before applying the techniques, so that important diagnoses such as malignancy are not being missed.

Script: Establish a baseline: pinch the web space between the thumb and index finger of the left hand to induce pain. Then do the same to the right hand. Make sure the patient is able to feel pain and the sensation is similar on both hands.

Pinch the web of the left hand to induce pain and apply one of the strategies while pinching the hand. Then pinch the web of the right hand and compare the two sides. If pain is less in the left hand, the strategy has worked. Identify which strategies work for the patient and then ask the patient to apply the strategy to the body part in pain.

<u>Attention on the pain:</u> 1) Focus your awareness on the pain until the sensation changes to something else. 2) Focus your awareness on your mind's reaction to the pain until the sensation changes.

<u>Attention away from the pain:</u> Focus your awareness on something other than the pain.

E.g., Subtract seven from a hundred and keep subtracting seven. Use Technique #1 and go to your imaginary safe place.

<u>Different perspective:</u> Imagine it's not your hand being pinched. Imagine you're stepping back and looking at the pain from some other place. Take a different perspective.

Different sensation: Imagine a different sensation at the site of pain. E.g., Imagine a tingling sensation from your thumb and index finger moving down to where you're pinching. Focus on the tingling sensation until the pain changes to a tingling sensation. E.g., Imagine numbness from your thumb and index finger moving down to where you're pinching. The numbness continues to spread across your hand. Soon all your fingers will feel numb. Now imagine all of your fingers are numb. Your entire hand is numb. Your wrist is numb. Pinch the other hand for comparison. If effective, imagine that both of your hands are numb in the area of a glove. You can apply the glove to any part of your body that is in pain. The numbness will spread from your hands into that body part so that it becomes numb.

TECHNIQUE #5: Imagining Cleansing

Description: A technique to help with repetitive washing, including showering or bathing and hand washing.

Rationale: Some patients may hold a feeling of disgust for their bodies, for example if they are victims of sexual assault. They need to understand that no amount of physical washing will be able to remove the psychological feeling of disgust, and that excessive washing can lead to dermatitis or other problems.

Script: Imagine soaking yourself in magical cleansing water. You can imagine a river, stream, holy water, or whatever feels right to you. Allow the cleansing power to enter all parts of your body, including all orifices. Believe that you are really clean.

TECHNIQUE #6: Auto-hypnosis using a Mirror

Description: Use a mirror to induce hypnosis.

Rationale: A strategy to help with feeling calmer and escaping emotional pain without using pathological self-soothing strategies, such as substances or dissociating. (See Chapter 9 Knowledge #10: Pathological Self-soothing / Addiction.)

Note: This is one of Milton Erickson's auto-hypnosis techniques.

Script: Set an alarm for twenty minutes. Get a mirror. Look at the mirror and empty your mind of any thoughts.

You know it is working if your sense of time changes (e.g., you lose track of time, or time passes quickly) or you feel like you are "out," or you wake up on your own after exactly twenty minutes.

Make sure you don't have food in your mouth; spit out your gum, so you don't choke. Make sure you're lying or sitting in a safe location, so you won't fall.

When you come back, notice how calm or focused you are.

TECHNIQUE #7: Shrinking Negative Emotions

Description: Using imagination to shrink negative emotions.

Rationale: Shrink negative emotions to make them more tolerable.

Script: Notice how ___ (e.g., anger) feels in your body. Notice what size it is. How big or small it is. What colour it is. What shape it is. What form it takes. How it moves. (Give me a nod when you have this.) Imagine moving that feeling outside of your body. Shrink the feeling to the size of a penny. Change its colour and shape to something calmer and softer. Change the direction of its movement. Now move this feeling back inside your body and notice how it feels. Notice how the sensation has changed.

TECHNIQUE #8: Imagining Success

Description: Imagining a successful future.

Rationale: This builds on Chapter 3 skills for fostering positive experiences. Help patients have a clearer image of their goal and feel that success is possible.

Script: Imagine the new life you want and what it would look like. Imagine reaching your goal. How good you look. How good you feel. Hear how good you sound. Become the person you would like to be.

TECHNIQUE #9: Healing the Inner Child

Description: Imagining positive experiences to heal one's inner child.

Rationale: Some patients have not experienced healthy parent-child interactions. By doing this exercise with the therapist, they can co-create what a healthy relationship looks like. This can now serve as a new template for healthy interactions, and can be used to repair attachment disorders. (See Chapter 8 Knowledge #1: Attachments.)

Note: Each scene can be done separately (about five minutes per scene) across appointments. Script 1 creates safety and Script 2 creates comfort. They can improve mood and sleep. Script 3 creates joy and can improve mood and self-esteem. Script 4 supports exploration and can improve self-esteem and foster exploration and self-development. Script 5 is about attunement and can help with emotional regulation and metacognitive skills. The concept of healing one's inner child developed out of Dr. Carl Jung's theories.

Script:

1) Picture yourself as a small child. Only you know best what your inner child really needs, so give your inner child what they need. You can imagine and re-imagine the scene however you like until it feels just right for you.

Now imagine a scene of you protecting your inner child. You create a perfectly safe environment for your inner child, being protective, but not overly protective. Vividly picture this scene.

Hear what you say to the child. It may be "you're safe," "I'll take care of you," or whatever phrase makes the most sense to you. Feel what it's like to protect this child and create a perfectly safe environment for them. (Give me a nod when you have this.) Describe the scene to me.

2) Let this scene fade and create another scene. Now imagine a scene of you comforting your inner child when they are emotionally upset. Only you know best how to comfort them. Imagine the way you soothe and comfort your inner child. Picture the physical closeness or the way you hold them. Hear what you say to the child to provide them with reassurance. It may be "It is okay to feel this way. It is reasonable to feel this way," or whatever phrase makes the most sense to you. Feel what it's like to comfort this child in all the right ways. (Give me a nod when you have this.) Describe the scene to me.

3) Let this scene fade and create another scene. Imagine yourself being with your inner child and consistently and openly expressing your joy at having this child. You are absolutely delighted with this child's being. They are the greatest source of happiness to you. There is nothing the child needs to do to please you. You are simply delighted in the child's being and you know they are wonderful. (Give me a nod when you have this.) Describe the scene to me.

4) Let this scene fade and create another scene. Imagine your inner child exploring and learning. You encourage and support the child to explore and discover in their own way. You are absolutely excited at what they learn and discover. You have no agenda for the child. You just want them to explore and discover in a relaxed and playful manner. You are fully supportive of the child's discovery and of them being truly who they want to be.

Your support helps to bring out the best in them. (Give me a nod when you have this.) Describe the scene to me.

5) Let this scene fade and create another scene. Imagine yourself being absolutely attuned to your inner child. You are curious about how your inner child is feeling, what they are thinking, what motivates their behaviour. You are interested in all their experiences and how they experience the world. You are attuned to their state of mind. You constantly wonder out loud how this child is feeling and thinking and what motivates their behaviour. You really see, hear, and know them. You are totally attuned and present with your inner child. (Give me a nod when you have this.) Describe the scene to me.

Let this scene fade. Now, check-in with your inner child and see what else they would like or need. Then give your inner child whatever they need. (Give me a nod when you have done so.) Describe the scene to me.

You may want to repeat: "Vividly picture this scene. Hear what you say to the child. Feel how he feels."

If the patient has difficulty imagining things, you can suggest things. The therapist and the patient co-create the imaginary scenes.

Things to provide soothing: physical proximity, the feeling of closeness, a sense of comfort, and verbal reassurance.

You might add, "Imagine the way you're holding this child."

Variation A: Imagining Ideal Parents

Description: Imagine having ideal parents.

Rationale: Patient and therapist co-create what having ideal parents looks like. This can help treat attachment disorders, foster metacognitive skills, emotional regulation, improves relationships, and self-development.

Note: Dr. Daniel Brown et al. created the Ideal Parents Figure (IPF) Protocol to create a new positive attachment representation.

Caveat: Some patients might find imagining ideal parents to be triggering because they realize what they have missed. Other patients might defend their parents. The clinician can say, "There's always room for improvement, and no parents are perfect." Healing the inner child tends to be easier to do.

Script: Just like the Healing the Inner Child technique, now imagine having ideal parents who help you feel safe, comfort you, are delighted in you, support you exploring, are attuned and present.

Stage 2 Skills

TECHNIQUE #9: Variation B: Letter to Inner Child

Description: Write a letter to the inner child and from the inner child to the adult self.

Rationale: Promote understanding and healing between the patient and their inner child.

Script: Write a letter to your inner child using your dominant hand. Then write a letter to your adult self from the perspective of the inner child using your non-dominant hand.

Sample response:

My dear child,

I want you to know that you're safe now. I am sorry for the horrible things that you suffered. You're so strong, brave, and smart. Know that you are wanted. Now you're heard and seen. You are a priority. You are not alone anymore. We'll get through this together. The adults failed you. You were just a child who needed love and affection. You did your best. We'll put the responsibility on those who were actually responsible.

Dear adult self,

I wish you had been here sooner. Reality has been cruel. Better late than never. It wasn't your fault.

TECHNIQUE #10: Imagining an Ideal Partner

Description: Using the qualities from Technique #9: Variation A: Imagining Ideal Parents to imagine having an equal partner with those qualities desired in an ideal parent.

Rationale: Sometimes people from abusive families end up in abusive relationships. People sometimes pick what's familiar over what's safe. This helps stop the unhealthy pattern.

Note: This is useful for both patients without partners and those with partners. For those without partners, once the patient has an idea of what to expect from a healthy relationship, they can search for a healthy relationship. For those in relationships, they can try to negotiate what they want with their partner. (See Chapter 6 on IPT.)

Script: Now imagine yourself in the future meeting an ideal partner. Imagine being in a relationship with someone who is an equal, and where you have a mutually gratifying relationship. You bring out the best in each other. This person has the qualities of an ideal parent figure, except that this time, this person is an equal. Imagine you and your partner providing each other with a safe environment. Imagine the comfort and reassurance you provide to each other. You are supportive of each other. You know that even when times are tough, you are there for each other and that you deeply love and care about each other. Imagine your qualities and the qualities of your ideal partner that make this a mutually gratifying relationship.

TECHNIQUE #11: Working with Nightmares

Description: Strategies to work with nightmares using a combination of mindfulness and imagination.

Rationale: Some people have recurrent nightmares; this is one strategy to gain mastery over them.

The different steps can be taught in different sessions.

Script:

Step One: Ask yourself: what's the difference between dreams and reality?

Use mindfulness: what's unreal about the dream?

E.g., Information about you, how places look, sound, feel, missing details, and lack of sense of smell/taste/touch.

When you're awake, ask yourself, "How do you know you're awake?"

At bedtime: rehearse facts about yourself, for example, your age, where you are, who's with you. This makes it easier for you to know you're in a dream when you're dreaming.

Step Two: Write down the nightmare.

What about the nightmare wakes you up? What's the conflict that's waking you up?

Include your feelings, thoughts, and information about the five senses.

Write down the changes you want to make to the nightmare.

E.g., Change the ending or the outcome.

Practice the new version of the dream.

Try different solutions until you find one that works.

For patients who get more diverse nightmare content, they can create something that would work for a variety of nightmares. It doesn't necessarily need to make sense.

E.g., Put a couple of friends into your dreams for support.

TECHNIQUE #12: Funeral of Broken Dreams

Description: Imaginary funeral for broken dreams.

Rationale: Helps the patient grieve and come to terms with what has been lost.

Script: We cannot change the past. Sometimes people wish that the past was different from what actually happened. There's a loss that has yet to be grieved. This may be grieving the childhood that you would have liked but never had, or wishing for wonderful parents, unlike the ones you had. Choose something that you wish to grieve for. Give me a nod when you have chosen something. Imagine holding a funeral for your broken dream. You acknowledge the grief associated with this. Imagine putting this dream into a coffin and burying it.

TECHNIQUE #13: Imagining a Timeline with Positive Experiences

Description: Putting positive life experiences onto an imaginary timeline.

Rationale: Help the patient have a sense of past, present, and future. Reinforce that life has ups and downs and nothing, no suffering, lasts forever.

Script: Imagine a timeline of your life. The timeline may be going from one side of you to the other side, or it may be going directly through you from front to back or any way that you would like to imagine it. The timeline represents the past, the present moment, and the future. Give me a nod when you're able to imagine this timeline. Go back as early as you can remember to a time when you were a young child. Think about your first positive experience. When you have this, give me a nod. Tell me about it. How does that make you feel? Where do you feel it in your body? I want you to hold on to this positive feeling. Give me a nod when you're ready to move to the next scene. Now continue along the timeline and think about your next positive experience.

Continue on along this timeline, identifying all the positive experiences that you have had. If any judgment comes up, just let it go. Give me a thumbs up when you have reached today. Now allow yourself to float above the timeline and take a look down. Look at the timeline going into your past, the spot that marks today, and the timeline continuing on representing the future. Notice all the positive experiences you have had over the years.

Variation A: Imagining a Timeline with Important Experiences

Description: Putting important life experiences (both positive and negative) onto an imaginary timeline.

Rationale: When the patient is able to tolerate the positive experiences, negative experiences can be added for a comprehensive timeline. This helps the patients integrate both positive and negative experiences into their life.

Note: Only do this if the patient feels ready and is able to tolerate negative emotions.

Script: Now that you have created an imaginary timeline with positive experiences, I want you to go back to the same timeline. This time, I want you to add in all the important experiences or impactful experiences even if they are negative experiences. Notice that life is full of ups and downs and nothing, no suffering, lasts forever. Notice your strength and how you have survived adversity.

Working with Traumatic Memories

TECHNIQUE #14: Boxing Difficult Memories

Description: Put difficult or traumatic memories into an imaginary box to save them for later.

Rationale: This may help some people regulate their emotions until they are able to face the reality of what happened to them.

Script: Imagine putting these memories into a box and closing the lid on it until you're ready to deal with the issue.

TECHNIQUE #15: Screens Method

Description: Project the traumatic memory onto an imaginary screen.

Rationale: The person can get some more emotional distance and it might help with self-regulation.

Script: Two Screens Method

Imagine two screens in front of you. Recall the difficult memory and project it onto one of the screens. On the other screen project a soothing image or scenario.

E.g., The patient imagines a friend comforting them on one screen or they imagine a bear attacking the perpetrator so that they feel safe and can express their anger.

Variation A: Add Ideal Parents to Screen Method

Description: Imagine watching the screen like viewing TV with ideal parents.

Script: Watch the screen with your ideal parents and imagine what they would say and the support that they would provide you.

TECHNIQUE #16: Adding Imaginary Elements

Description: Add imaginary elements to the traumatic memory.

Rationale: This can make the memory more tolerable, and help the patient get unstuck from that loop.

Script: Try adding imaginary elements to the traumatic memory. You can try the following, whichever works for you:

- Imagine what you would like to have been able to do.

- See it in black and white.
- Play it backward.
- Change the voice into a funny voice.
- Change the smell.

Summary

Hypnotic techniques can help patients relax. They can be used to treat anxiety or insomnia by creating safe spaces and adjusting emotional intensity. Given the mind-body connection, relaxation can also reduce physical problems such as IBS, sexual dysfunction, chronic pain, and high blood pressure. Hypnotic techniques can reduce feelings of disgust and improve obsessive compulsive behaviour. Auto-hypnosis can help patients escape from emotional pain without using pathological self-soothing strategies such as substances or dissociating. By imagining success, patients can have a clearer image of their goal and feel that success is possible.

Healing the Inner Child and Imagining Ideal Parents are powerful techniques that repair attachment disorders and create new templates for healthy interactions. Qualities of the imagined ideal parents can help the patient visualize an ideal partner, leading them to search for a healthier relationship or negotiate what they want with their partner.

Imagination can treat PTSD symptoms by addressing nightmares and making traumatic memories more tolerable. The funeral of broken dreams helps patients grieve and process emotions. When patients imagine a timeline they can get a sense of the past, present, and future and understand that suffering is transient. Reflecting on both positive and negative experiences helps them have a more well-rounded perspective that life has ups and downs. The use of imagination opens patients up to new possibilities, including engaging in new behaviours, thoughts, and feelings.

CHAPTER 5:
Cognitive Behavioural Therapy (CBT)

Dr. Aaron Beck created CBT in the 1960s. It is a well-researched and commonly used psychotherapy technique, but over time, new psychotherapy techniques have been developed from the classic CBT. (See Chapter 7: Dialectical Behaviour Therapy (DBT) / Beyond the Classic CBT.) This chapter covers the classic CBT.

CBT is the gold standard for treating anxiety disorders (including generalized anxiety disorder, phobia, panic disorder, social anxiety, agoraphobia) and anxiety related disorders (OCD, PTSD). See below for the Anxiety Model. In addition, CBT can be used to treat depression, bipolar disorder, BPD, eating disorders, insomnia, addiction, psychosis (reduces intensity of delusions), and sexual disorders. Given the link between mental health and physical health, CBT can also improve physical health conditions such as IBS, chronic pain, fibromyalgia, and chronic fatigue syndrome. (See Chapter 9 Knowledge #12: Trauma's Impact on Physical Body and Disease.)

The concepts of cognitive dissonance and ambivalence help to explain how CBT works. Using the patient's own ambivalence and working with different parts or aspects of self can help motivate the patient to change. This chapter also covers exposure treatment and response prevention, which reduces anxiety by changing behaviour.

The ABCs of CBT

Affect (emotion), **B**ehaviour, and **C**ognition (thoughts)

These three things affect one another. The patient can get into a negative feedback loop where each component of the ABC exacerbates the underlying problem.

Sample response:

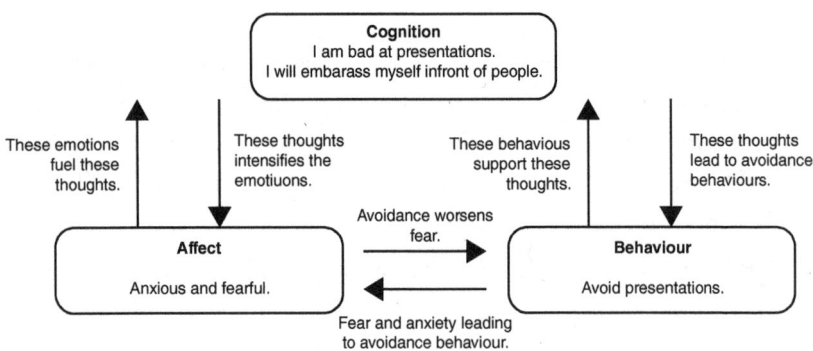

Figure 2: CBT

By changing one component of the ABCs, the negative feedback loop can be interrupted and improved.

CBT targets:

- Unhelpful behaviour that maintains this cycle.
- Unhelpful cognition that maintains this cycle.

CBT Analyzes:

- **A**ntecedent, **B**elief (cognition), **C**onsequence (see Technique #5.)
- **A**ntecedent, **B**ehaviour, **C**onsequence (see Technique #13.)

Anxiety Model

Although the Diagnostic and Statistical Manual of Mental Disorders 5 (DSM-5) moved OCD and PTSD out of anxiety disorders and into their own section, it is still helpful to think about the relationship between them.

This helps conceptualize the relationship.

Continuous Hyperarousal

- Generalized anxiety disorder (GAD): Worries are generally realistic but excessive. Patients overestimate risks and underestimate coping ability. Patients fear uncertainty.
- Obsessive-compulsive behaviour:
    - Obsessions: Make the patient anxious, triggers can be internal (e.g., thoughts, images) or external (e.g., contaminated objects).
    - Compulsion: What the patient does to avoid or eliminate the danger/anxiety. It includes behaviour (e.g., cleaning) and cognitive compulsions (e.g., counting, mental review). Compulsion is used to cope with anxiety. The compulsions can be excessive of what's functional (cleaning) or non-functional (rituals).
    - The patient's appraisal of the obsessions and compulsion also perpetuates the hyperarousal. E.g., Thoughts are harmful. If I think about it, then I'm going to do it or it's going to happen (thought-action fusion).
    - Fear of uncertainty, perfectionism, need to control, taking too much responsibility.

Episodic Hyperarousal

- Phobia: Fear of an external stimulus.
- Panic disorder: Fear of internal cues or internal states and worry that it means they're dying or going crazy. Fear of losing control.
- Social anxiety: Fear of humiliation and negative evaluations.
- Agoraphobia: Panic and avoidance of being trapped somewhere during an episode.

Hyperarousal in PTSD
- Continuous hypervigilance, like GAD.
- Episodic hyperarousal:
    - External triggers: Sight, sound, smell, physical sensation, people, situation, etc.
    - Internal triggers: Thoughts, emotion, memories, bodily sensations, etc.
- Avoidance of triggers.
- Fear of the memory, emotions, and parts or self-states.

Cognitive Dissonance

Cognitive dissonance occurs when people's beliefs, values, feelings, or behaviours don't align. This creates mental discomfort. People will try to reduce this discomfort by changing their beliefs or justifying their actions.

Stage 1 Skills

Cognition

TECHNIQUE #1: Cognitive Distortions / Hot Thoughts

Description: Identifying hot thoughts.

Rationale: Help patients to identify hot thoughts and what bothers them.

Script: Here is a list of hot thoughts, their description, and examples. Let's review them together. I want you to write down your hot thoughts and bring them to our next clinic.
- All or Nothing Thinking: Seeing only extremes or seeing situations as black or white.

- E.g., Either I'm the best mother in the world or I'm a terrible mother.
- Shoulds: "Should" is negative. It implies failure, reinforces judgment, and focuses on the past as opposed to the present or the future.
    - E.g., I should have done better.
- Jumping to Conclusions: Reaching conclusions when there is no evidence to support them.
    - Mind Reading: Acting as though you know what other people are thinking.
        - E.g., I know she hates me.
    - Fortune telling: Predicting the future.
        - E.g., This will only end in failure.
- Mental filter: Only paying attention to one type of evidence.
    - Discounting the Positives: Focusing on the negatives while ignoring the positives.
        - E.g., I can't ever get it right.
- Labelling: Characterizing ourselves or others.
    - E.g., I am stupid.
- Double Standard: Holding oneself to a different standard than other people.
    - E.g., It is okay for others to get help for mental illness, but not okay if I do so.
- Magnification / Catastrophizing / Blowing Things Out of Proportion: Making a small thing much larger than it realistically is.
    - E.g., If I don't do well on the presentation tomorrow, my career is over.
- Emotional Reasoning: I feel a certain way and therefore it must be true.
    - E.g., Those people make me feel nervous. They must be out to get me.

- Blaming: Taking too much responsibility for things outside of your control or blaming others for something that was your responsibility.
    - E.g., If anyone in my family gets ill, it is all my fault.
- Over-Generalizing: Applying one outcome in a broader range of scenarios than needed.
    - E.g., My friend did not want to hang out with me today. He never wants to hang out with me again.
- Magical Thinking: Believing things will all be better when ___.
    - E.g., Everything will be better if I lose weight.
- Thought-action Fusion: If I think about it, then I'm going to do it, or it's going to happen.
    - E.g., I had a thought about hurting my boss. I am going to end up hurting him.

TECHNIQUE #2: Therapist to Identify and Challenge Hot Thoughts

Description: Therapist to identify and challenge a patient's hot thoughts.

Rationale: By identifying and challenging hot thoughts, the patient may become more aware of them. Reframing them can reduce the emotional intensity.

Script:

Patient's Hot Thoughts	Therapist Challenges Hot Thoughts
Either I'm the best mother in the world or I'm a terrible mother.	Are there people who are just average mothers who try but don't always get it right?

Patient's Hot Thoughts	Therapist Challenges Hot Thoughts
I should have done better.	Is this a realistic expectation?
I know she hates me. This will only end in failure.	How do you know that?
I can't ever get it right.	Are there times you do get it right? You showed up to therapy today and that's one right thing you're doing towards your wellbeing.
I am stupid.	What would a friend say?
It is okay for others to get help for mental illness, but not okay if I do so.	If you had a friend who's struggling with mental health difficulties, what would you do or say to him?
If I don't do well on the presentation tomorrow, my career is over.	What makes you say this? What evidence supports this? What evidence does not support this?
Those people make me feel nervous. They must be out to get me.	What else might be making you feel nervous about these people?
If anyone in my family gets ill, it is my fault.	Who else might be responsible for this? How much responsibility do you think each of your family members has?
My friend did not want to hang out with me today. He never wants to hang out with me again.	How do you know it's about you? Are there other reasons that he may not want to hang out today? Did he tell you that he never wanted to hang out again? Is that how he is with everyone?

Patient's Hot Thoughts	Therapist Challenges Hot Thoughts
Everything will be better if I lose weight.	Can you give me examples of what you believe would be better when you've lost weight? What makes you believe this?
I had a thought about hurting my boss. I am going to end up hurting him.	Can you try thinking about winning the lottery and see if that is going to happen?

TECHNIQUE #3: Myths About Thoughts

Description: There are myths about thoughts just as there are myths about emotions. (See Chapter 2 Technique #2: Addressing Fears and Myths about Emotions.) Explore myths about thoughts to help create distance between the self and the thoughts.

Rationale: Putting some distance between oneself and thoughts helps patients tolerate distressing thoughts better.

Script: I am going to read out some statements. Tell me whether you believe them to be true or false, or the extent to which you believe this on a scale of one to ten, ten being you fully believe this.

Each of the following is a myth about thoughts. This means they are untrue statements that some people might believe. Let's go through each one and discuss it.

- You are your thoughts.
- Always trust your thoughts. They are truths.
- If you have thought about it, it's going to happen or you will do it.

TECHNIQUE #4: Creating Distance from Hot Thoughts

Description: Strategies to create distance between patients and their thoughts.

Rationale: Help patients tolerate distressing thoughts better.

Script: I am going to give you some strategies that will help you create distance between yourself and your thoughts. I want you to pick at least one of them and try it.

When you are having a hot thought, I want you to add, "I am having the thought of…" or simply say to yourself, "Thank you, brain, for the thought."

You can also change the hot thought by singing it, saying it in a funny voice, saying it very quickly or very slowly.

Which of these strategies do you want to try?

TECHNIQUE #5: Antecedent, Belief, Consequence

Description: Identify the ABC of CBT for a belief.

Rationale: Help patients recognize the connection between their beliefs and the consequences.

Script: Let's go over an example. A person is going to a party. He thinks he's uncool and unpopular and that people don't like hanging around him. This leads him to act awkwardly around others, which in turn makes other people feel awkward and uncomfortable around him. He then leaves the party early. This is what the ABC chart for belief looks like for him.

If he thinks instead that he's cool and enjoys socializing, he might act more confidently and comfortably around others. This may make others enjoy being around him. Can you think of an example where one of your negative beliefs leads to an undesired consequence?

Antecedent (Situation)	Belief (Cognition / Hot Thoughts)	Consequences
Going to a party.	I am uncool and unpopular. People don't like hanging out with me.	Act awkwardly around other people, which in turn makes other people feel awkward and uncomfortable around me. Leave the party early.

TECHNIQUE #6: Getting to the Core Belief

Description: Explore the hot thought.

Rationale: Identify the hot thoughts and core beliefs that are really bothering the person.

Script: What does that say about you? What would happen if you actually did terribly?

Sample response:

Situation	Thoughts
I need to give a presentation tomorrow.	I will do terribly on the presentation tomorrow. I'll embarrass myself in front of my colleagues. I'll lose my job and no one will ever want to hire me. If I don't do well on the presentation tomorrow, my career is over. I am a failure.

TECHNIQUE #7: Facts Supporting, Facts Against

Description: Find facts that support and refute the hot thoughts using the example above.

Rationale: Identifying facts helps to tease out what are facts versus judgments. This will help patients move towards a more balanced perspective.

Note: See Chapter 2 Technique #4: Judgments versus Facts.

Script: What are facts that support your belief?

What are facts that do not support your belief?

Remember facts are things that you can prove. It might help to think like a lawyer presenting evidence to the judge.

Is this a fact or a judgment or a habitual belief?

Facts Supporting	Facts Against
I did poorly on my last presentation and my boss gave me negative feedback.	I did not lose my job. The last one was my first presentation for this company and I've learned from it.

Other things to consider: Is this information reliable? Are these relevant factors? Is this an interpretation of the event or a fact?

TECHNIQUE #8: Locus of Control

Description: People who have an internal locus of control feel they control their own life and outcome, while those who have an external locus of control feel other people and situations control their life and the outcome. People exist on a spectrum. Where they fit depends on how much they feel their locus of control is internal versus external.

Rationale: Shifting the locus of control from external to internal can help patients feel more in control and help them to have a sense of self-agency.

Script: Instead of thinking "It was an easy exam," give yourself some credit and remind yourself, "I studied hard and I prepared for it."

TECHNIQUE #9: Assigning Responsibility

Description: Assigning an appropriate amount of responsibility.

Rationale: Help patients think about who else has responsibility, and what part of the situation the patients might actually have control over.

Script: I want to go back to your statement, "If anyone in my family gets ill, it is my fault."

How much responsibility do you think each person in your family has to protect each other from getting ill?

Sample response: At the start, the patient assigns himself 100% of the responsibility for preventing family members from getting ill. After the discussion, the patient assigns himself 35%, his wife 35%, his parents 20%, and his children 10%.

TECHNIQUE #10: Cumulative Probability

Description: Assign the appropriate probabilities.

Rationale: Help patients be more realistic about the probabilities of a bad outcome.

Script: You were very upset and anxious when you stepped on the sticky floor at work. You were worried that you might catch a disease and die. I want you to assign probability to each of the events, then multiply the probability to get the cumulative probability.

Event	Probability
It was someone's bodily fluid. e.g., urine (and not juice or something else).	1/2
The bodily fluid contains communicable disease.	1/10
I contract a disease from contact with the floor while wearing shoes.	1/100
The disease is a serious illness.	1/10
I die from the disease despite medical treatment.	1/10

Cumulative Probability	1x1x1x1/2x10x100x10x10= 1/200,000

Affect

TECHNIQUE #11: Noticing the Emotion and Situation

Description: Patients explore the emotion and the situation surrounding the emotional experience.

Rationale: Help patients bring awareness to the emotion and situation so they can begin to work on the emotion. Identify how intense the emotion is, so it can be re-rated after the CBT exercise.

Note: See Chapter 2 Technique #1: Teaching Language for Emotions, and Technique #3: Identify Intensity of Emotions.

Script: You wanted to work on your anxiety. I want you to keep track of situations where you are feeling anxious.

Ask yourself: When do I feel anxious? What is going on that is making me feel so anxious?

Now rate the intensity of the emotions from zero to a hundred.

Sample response:

Situation	Emotions and Intensity (0-100)
I need to give a presentation tomorrow.	Anxious: 90.

TECHNIQUE #12: Adding Body Sensation

Description: Explore the body sensation associated with the emotion. Combining techniques from Chapters 1 and 5.

Rationale: This is helpful for patients who are psychosomatic or have difficulty identifying their emotions. Help patients explore their internal bodily sensations and not fear them.

Script: What does anxiety feel like to you? Where in the body do you feel it?

Sample response: Anxiety feels like tightness in my shoulders, neck, and chest.

Behaviour

TECHNIQUE #13: Antecedent, Behaviour, Consequence

Description: Identify the ABC of CBT for a behaviour.

Rationale: Help patients recognize the connection between their behaviour and the consequences.

Script: Let's go over an example. A patient did not get the appointment time he wanted. He started yelling and swearing at the receptionist. The consequence was he got a warning letter that he could be terminated from the practice if this continues. He still did not get the appointment time he wanted. This is what the ABC chart for behaviour looks like for him.

If instead he had asked to be put on a cancellation list or stated a reason why he needed an earlier appointment, he could have seen another practitioner sooner.

Can you think of an example where one of your behaviours led to an undesired consequence?

Antecedent (Situation)	Behaviour	Consequences
Not being able to get the appointment time I wanted.	Yelling and swearing at the receptionist.	Getting a warning letter that I could be terminated from the practice if this continues. I did not get the appointment time I wanted.

TECHNIQUE #14: Rewarding Desired Behaviour

Description: Reward desired behaviour, don't reward undesired behaviours. Reward behaviours that are close to the target behaviour so that the patients move closer to the target behaviour.

Rationale: Rewarding a behaviour increases the likelihood of the behaviour recurring. Behaviour is shaped by experiences. People can change behaviour.

Script: I expect therapy to be helpful, so we will review your progress every three months to make sure you're making gains. I will continue therapy only if this is helpful to you.

(A patient gets to continue therapy if they are making progress, instead of terminating therapy when they're doing well. Reward progress.)

E.g., A patient is yelling. The therapist covers his ears and says, "It's too loud. It hurts my ears." When the patient calms down, the therapist uncovers his ears and says, "Thank you for using your quiet voice." This helps patients gain awareness of their actions and rewards the good behaviour of using a quiet voice to get the therapist's attention.

E.g., A child is sitting quietly. The therapist rewards the behaviour by saying, "Thank you for sitting so nicely." They can give additional incentives by saying, "If you continue to sit this nicely, I'll give you a sticker at the end of our appointment."

TECHNIQUE #15: Behaviour Activation

Description: Using behaviour to change mood or cognition.

Rationale: People have difficulty getting things started, but once they do, it is much easier to keep going.

Note: This book uses the principle of spending five minutes a day to learn psychotherapy techniques.

Script: You mentioned that you are feeling very depressed and you are doing very little. You have thought about doing exercises, but you haven't done so. I want you to exercise for five minutes a day. Do you think you would be able to set aside five minutes a day to do something towards your recovery?

Combined

TECHNIQUE #16: Putting it Together

Description: Patients track and complete the CBT recording. They come up with a balanced perspective, then re-rate the emotion intensity using the example above.

Rationale: Once patients have learned the different components, they can start challenging their own hot thoughts. Coming up with a balanced perspective that's supported by evidence will often reduce emotional distress.

Note: See Chapter 3 Technique #4: Reframing.

Script: Now that you have learned the various components, let's put them together. I want you to keep track of situations that bring up the negative emotion you want to work on and complete the chart. Now combine the facts supporting and facts against the hot thought and come up with a new, more balanced perspective. Once you have a more balanced perspective, re-rate the intensity of your emotion. Let's review the chart together at the next visit.

Situation	Thoughts	Emotions and Intensity (0-100)	Body Sensation
I need to give a presentation tomorrow.	I will do terribly on the presentation tomorrow. I'll embarrass myself in front of my colleagues. I'll lose my job and no one will ever want to hire me.	Anxious: 90.	Tightness in shoulders, neck, and chest.

Facts Supporting	Facts Against	Balanced Perspective	Re-rate Affect and Intensity
I did poorly on my last presentation and my boss gave me negative feedback.	I did not lose my job. The last one was my first presentation for this company and I've learned from it.	I did poorly on the last presentation, but I learned from it and I probably won't lose my job.	Anxiety: 65.

TECHNIQUE #17: Ambivalence / Working with Parts

Description: Working with ambivalence or different parts of a patient.

Rationale: If the therapist tells a patient to stop a behaviour, the conflict becomes between the patient and the therapist. However, if the therapist allows the patient to explore within themselves for the part of them that wants to quit versus the part that wants to continue the behaviour, the conflict becomes internal.

Note: Dr. Richard Schwartz created the Internal Family Systems Therapy.

Script: 1) One part of you feels smoking is damaging your health and wants to stop. The other part of you gets something out of continuing this behaviour. This is a deep conflict within yourself. Allow the different parts of yourself to talk to each other. All parts of you have something important to say. I want you to listen to all of them. What's each part of you trying to tell you? Learn from it.

2) Patient: I've tried everything and nothing worked.

Therapist: Is there a part of you that's blocking you from getting better? It can be scary to get better and that part of you might be keeping you safe.

Patient: I guess there's a part of me that doesn't want to deal with all these intense emotions.

Therapist: There's a part of you trying to keep you safe from feeling intense emotions. Can you work with that part of you to allow you to feel some emotions? (Go back to Chapter 2 Technique #2: Addressing Fears and Myths about Emotions and see Stage 1 Skills for emotional regulation strategies.)

TECHNIQUE #18: Working with the Self-Critical Part

Description: Work with the self-critical part or voice.

Rationale: Help patients recognize and work with the self-critical part.

Script: Where is the negative, self-critical voice coming from? (Did it remind the patient of one of their parents who was critical?)

Where is it located in the body?

What would happen if you didn't have that critical voice?

How has the critical voice helped you? Instead of adding more self-blame on top of self-blame, acknowledge and thank it for what it has done previously. Let the critical voice know that this is no longer necessary. Its job is done as the present is different from the past.

Stage 2 Skills

Exposure Treatment:

TECHNIQUE #19: Story on Fear and Avoidance

Description: Tell patients a story about fear and avoidance.

Rationale: Help patients learn from the story and relate it to their own struggles with fear and avoidance.

Script: I am going to read you a story.

Ms. J parks her car in the parking lot. Every time she crosses the barrier gate, she gets very afraid. She worries that the bar will accidentally come down on her car. She started coming in early to find street parking so that she won't have to park in the parking lot. One day, she couldn't find street parking and had to use the parking lot. The barrier gate came down on her car, just as she had feared. It left a yellow scratch on the roof of her car. However, she stopped being afraid and started parking in the parking lot again. She previously had worried that the gate would go through the windshield and stab her, dent the roof of the car and crush her, or she'd break it and get charged with property destruction, but none of these happened.

Think about the story. What does it tell you about fear and avoidance?

Sample response: Avoiding something might make the fear worse. By facing her fear, she learned that it was not as bad as she had imagined.

TECHNIQUE #20: Exposure Treatment

Description: Expose patients to what they fear and prevent the avoidance / escape behaviour.

Rationale: Exposure treatment helps patients learn from the situation, be present, and be able to tolerate the feelings. Patients learn that anxiety is an emotion and it is not dangerous. They also learn that they can make choices and change their behaviour. Help them to be able to function despite the anxiety and reach their goals.

Note: Avoidance extends to memories as well. The point of exposure treatment isn't to blast patients with their traumatic memories, nor to desensitize or habituate patients. Some patients never reach habituation. The more avoidance, the more likely exposure treatment would be helpful. It doesn't need to be hierarchical, but does need to promote new learning and be at a distress level that the patient can tolerate without engaging in avoidance / escape behaviour. Life is full of "exposures."

What to expose the patient to depends on what they fear and are avoiding.

GAD: Expose them to what they are worried about. Think of the worst-case scenario.

Alternate exposure with Stage 1 Skills such as relaxation and mindfulness, so the patient can tolerate the experience and not avoid it.

OCD: Expose them and prevent the escape response. Prevent the ritual.

E.g., Patient is worried that she will hurt a child, even though that's never happened. The exposure could be to the child.

Panic: Exposure to intensified bodily sensation / state of mind.

Phobia: Exposure to the feared object. This can be imaginary exposure.

Script: You have a fear of using public washrooms.

What's the worst thing that might happen?

Patient: I will catch a disease and die.

Therapist: Let's do a cumulative probability exercise. (See Technique #15: Assign Probability.)

Patient: I think public washrooms are gross.

Therapist: Let's reframe it as I'm noticing the thought that "this is gross." (See Technique #4: Create Distance with Hot Thoughts.)

Exposure: Use a public washroom. (If this is too much, go to a public washroom and touch the walls.)

Response prevention: Don't wash your hands until you're ready to eat.

TECHNIQUE #21: Meaning of the Exposure Treatment

Description: Find out how the exposure aligns with the patient's goals and values.

Rationale: Find out why the patient is wanting to do the exposure and the meaning behind it to serve as motivation. To achieve lasting change it is important that this is meaningful.

Note: See Chapter 3 Technique #7: Values.

Script: What is meaningful about the exposure? How does doing this fit in with your values and goals?

Sample response: If I can use the public washroom, I can go out and be around my friends. My friends are important to me. I'll also feel good about myself.

TECHNIQUE #22: Combining Exposure Treatment with Mindfulness

Description: Use mindfulness skills during exposure treatment. Notice thoughts and sensations and explore appraisal.

Rationale: Help patients observe and reflect on the situation. Mindfulness can help reduce distress.

Note: This combines techniques from Chapters 1 and 5. Try to keep a collaborative spirit in exposure exercises. Help patients be self-compassionate about the exposure. Provide support, but not reassurance. Teach patients to self-reassure.

Script: What's showing up for you? What thoughts are you noticing? What bodily sensations are you noticing?

What did you learn from the experience?

What surprised you?

Summary

CBT helps to identify hot thoughts and challenge core negative beliefs. By examining the facts, patients come up with a more balanced perspective. The CBT record helps the patient see the connection between thoughts, feelings, behaviours, and body sensations. Through the use of cognitive dissonance, changing one of these can change the other. CBT also brings attention to the connection between a situation, behaviour, and the consequences. The patient can use this knowledge to change their behaviours. When desired behaviours are rewarded, their frequency increases. Using behaviour activation, and practising the new behaviour five minutes a day, patients can be motivated to change and create improved habits. Behaviour activation can also be used to help therapists learn new psychotherapy techniques.

Working with ambivalence and parts of self can also motivate patients to change. Exposure therapy is another powerful tool. It changes emotions by changing the behaviour and is especially effective when used to address anxiety disorders.

CHAPTER 6:
Interpersonal Therapy (IPT)

Humans are relational creatures. Relationships are important for physical and mental health and wellbeing. They help people meet their physical, emotional, and social needs.

Dr. Gerald Klerman and Dr. Myrna Weissman created IPT in the 1960s. IPT can be used to treat a wide range of disorders, including mood disorders, eating disorders, and chronic fatigue. It also addresses stressors brought on by life transitions, such as deaths, births, and new roles. Patients with personality disorders are relationally challenged and will benefit from improved interpersonal skills. Use of IPT can improve the situation when a lack of interpersonal skills interferes with functioning or when interpersonal conflicts drive symptoms.

Trauma can leave the patient feeling isolated and fearing others. Therefore, patients with PTSD can also benefit from IPT, because it helps the patient focus on the present, engage socially, experience positive interpersonal interactions, and learn to trust people again rather than dwell on past traumatic experiences. Patients also learn to emotionally regulate and communicate their feelings and needs in a healthy way. They learn to set boundaries and give constructive feedback, which helps them to be consistently assertive instead of alternating between avoidance and aggression.

Goals of IPT

- Improve function and reduce symptoms.
- Repair and strengthen good relationships.
- Expand and improve social support. Find healthy relationships: choose the right people and act appropriately.
- Build meaningful emotional connections with others.

- Help the patient feel seen, heard, and understood. Improve communication skills so the patient can communicate their feelings, thoughts, and needs.
- Problem-solve through what the patient can change and accept and what cannot be changed. Grieve what is lost.
- Help the patient gain a sense of mastery and be successful in navigating interpersonal relationships and fulfilling their social role. This helps with self-esteem and aids the patient in learning to expect positive things.
- Separate the past from the present. This includes exploring and challenging problematic behaviours that were previously helpful, but are no longer useful.

Society and Culture

Culture and society set up expectations regarding relationships and roles. They affect how the patients see and interpret the world. They are incorporated into patients' identities. Fulfilling social roles and finding a sense of belonging and purpose affect their self-esteem. Society and culture can provide support and connection, and help with healing. The therapist needs to be sensitive to the patient's social and cultural context, and link issues and symptoms back to them.

Ingredients:

- Self-awareness
- Perspective-taking
- Emotional regulation skills
- Communication skills
- Negotiation skills

Consideration

Participating in group therapy can help the patients make connections with other patients and feel that they are not alone in their struggles. Peer-to-peer support may also have similar benefits.

If the patient is a child, teach the parent (or whoever is the primary support for the child) parenting skills and get the parent involved with therapy. A therapist can role-model and coach caregivers. Sometimes the parent may need treatment themselves. The child who is struggling may be a "canary in the coal mine," and the family needs to heal together.

A patient can also heal by finding or building a community where they belong and have social supports. E.g., A refugee in a new country can benefit from finding a new community.

Stage 1 Skills

Information Gathering

TECHNIQUE #1: Exploring Patients' Social Networks

Description: Explore which people are important in the patient's life.

Rationale: Gathering information will help identify the patient's problems and explore their strengths and supports.

Note: Pay attention to what makes the patient want to seek help now. The patient may have difficulty navigating and coping with changes, loss, and conflicts.

Script: Who are the important people in your life? Think about your family, friends, and colleagues.

Who do you see on most days?

Who do you live with?

Who do you turn to when you're upset?

Who do you turn to when you need help?

Who improves your symptoms? Who worsens them?

TECHNIQUE #2: Closeness Circle

Description: Display the people who are important in the patient's life in multiple concentric circles.

Rationale: Help them understand and represent graphically the people who are close to them.

Script: I want you to put the people who are important in your life on the closeness circle. In the smallest circle next to you, write down the people who are closest to you.

Sample response: The patient is the closest to her husband who is in the intimate circle. She's good friends with Basil and her mother, whom she places in the second circle. She has Kent, a supportive colleague, and Rosemary, another friend.

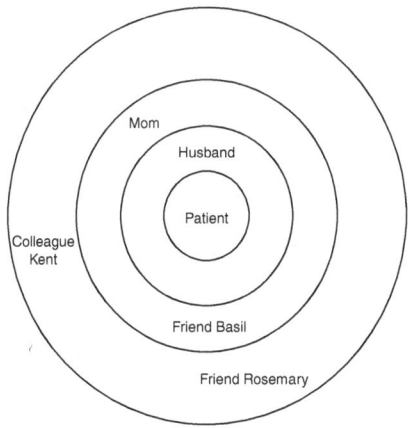

Figure 3a: Closeness Circle

PART I: TECHNIQUES

TECHNIQUE #3: How has the Relationship Changed

Description: Exploring changes in relationships.

Rationale: Times of change can be stressful and may be contributing to the patient's symptoms. There may be losses that haven't been grieved. There may be conflict that needs to be explored and problems solved. Drawing the closeness circle and visualizing how relationships have changed help the therapist obtain information.

Note: It is easier to look at the closeness circle and ask the patient to draw out how the relationship has changed.

Script: Which relationships have changed? How have the changes affected you? When did the change happen? What do you think triggered the change? How do you feel about the change? What does the change say about you?

Sample response: Since my father died, my mother has been relying on me more. However, my husband is finding her involvement to be intrusive, and we are fighting a lot. My friend Rosemary lost her father a few years ago, and she has been more supportive. I find that she and I are getting closer together.

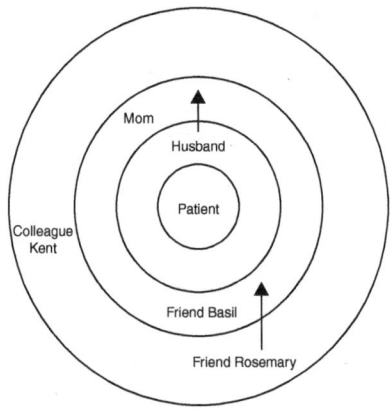

Figure 3b: Closeness Circle Change

TECHNIQUE #4: Self-Awareness

Description: Help patients to self-reflect on their goals.

Rationale: Help the patients identify what they want and explore their intentions.

Script: What would you like to see in the relationship? How do you want those people to respond to you? Why is this important to you?

Identifying Issues

TECHNIQUE #5: Exploring the Issue

Description: Explore the patient's understanding of the issue.

Rationale: Explore who, what, when, and where, nonjudgmentally first. Then help the patient to self-reflect on the conversation and how it is related to the problematic outcome. There may be difficulty with communication because of the problems involved in understanding each other or expressing feelings and needs.

Note: Conflicts tend to arise from differences in expectations and values, difficulty with communication, or broken (implicit or explicit) agreements.

Script: What happened? What did you say? What was the other person's response? What was the outcome?

How did you feel? What was going through your mind?

What would you like to communicate? What do you think the other person understood? How do you think the other person felt? What do you think the other person wanted? Why do you think the other person responded this way?

What is the underlying problem? What do you think caused the problem? How much of an impact does this problem have?

How did this affect your relationship? How long do you think this issue will last?

TECHNIQUE #6: Exploring Expectations

Description: Explore the patient's expectations.

Rationale: Help the patient reflect on the expectation and consider the other person's perspective.

Script: What's your expectation? How have you shared this expectation? Do you think the other person understood the expectation? Is this a reasonable and realistic expectation for the other person? What motivates you to meet this expectation? What do you think motivates the other person to meet this expectation? Is this a reciprocal relationship?

Communication

TECHNIQUE #7: Turn-Taking / Speaker Object

Description: The patient takes turns with the other person while communicating.

Rationale: Communication is a two-way street. Each person needs to have a chance to express themselves and be heard.

Note: This technique is for the patient who talks over the other person or vice versa.

Script: It sounds like when you and your husband have an argument, you are yelling over each other. Neither of you feels heard. Both of you feel that you don't have the chance to express what you need to say.

One of the most important rules of communication is turn-taking. Only one person talks at a time. You need to wait for the other person to finish before you start talking, and vice versa. One of the things you can try is using a speaker object. This is an object that you both agree on; whoever is holding it gets to speak. Once the person is done speaking, the object is passed to the other person, so that they can start speaking. Whoever is not holding the speaker object has to listen.

For example, you and your husband can use a tissue box as a speaker object and agree on the rule. Try it and let me know how it goes.

TECHNIQUE #8: "I" Statement

Description: The patients reframe statements into "I" statements.

Rationale: "I" statements help the patients communicate their feelings and their needs.

Script: Instead of saying "You always make such a mess," reframe it as an "I" statement. For example, you can say, "I feel angry when you leave the dirty dishes on the table after you have eaten. I would like you to put the dirty dishes in the sink after you are done." Now, you try another example.

TECHNIQUE #9: Beyond What is Said

Description: Be mindful that communication is more than what is said.

Rationale: Communication is also how it is said and what is not said. It includes non-verbal communication.

Script: Practice what you want to say in front of a mirror, or record it to see how you look and hear how you sound. Notice the tone of your voice. What does the tone convey? Does it match what you want to convey? Try changing the tone and notice the difference. Notice the way you stand, where you place your arms, your hands, your legs, your feet. Notice your body language, whether your arms are crossed or open. Try to avoid passive-aggressive postures, body language, and tone of voice, such as eye rolling. Think about and practice leaning in towards the person with open arms and body posture to show interest. Think about what the other person might hear or how the other person might interpret it. Try it at home then we will practice it together in the office.

TECHNIQUE #10: Active Listening

Description: Teach the patients to actively listen to the other person by validating and summarizing the other person's statements.

Rationale: To meet the other person's need of wanting to be heard and understood. It helps to make sure that everyone is on the same page. The patient can appreciate the thought and the intent, but not the action. Summarizing can convey empathy and understanding. Understanding is not equal to agreeing.

Script: Pay attention and gather information while the other person is talking.

Try using these phrases:

"I hear you."

"Let me make sure I heard you correctly." Then summarize what you heard.

"Slow down. Let me just summarize what you said."

"Just to clarify…"

"I can see how you would feel frustrated."

TECHNIQUE #11: Practicing Self-Disclosures and Small Favours

Description: Each person slowly discloses more of themselves and practices asking for small favours in order to build trust.

Rationale: To build trust and emotional safety.

Note: These are small things where the patient feels the outcome is inconsequential. The patient needs to be okay with having someone say no, and not feel rejected or upset.

Script: Practice giving small things: E.g., I'm going downtown today. Is there anything you would like me to pick up while I'm there?

Practice asking for small things: E.g., I would like to go out for a walk tomorrow and I would love some company. Are you available?

Practice self-disclosure: E.g., I used to enjoy sneaking out to the beach when my parents weren't around.

TECHNIQUE #12: Giving Feedback

Description: Give timely and strategic feedback.

Rationale: Help the patient give feedback strategically. Avoid the silent treatment.

Script: It is important that you give feedback to the other person in a timely manner so that they can improve. This helps to prevent problems and emotions from building up. Start with something you appreciate and another thing you feel the other person can improve on. Try to focus on the positives.

I appreciate your thoughts and your good intentions. At the same time, I just want...

E.g., I appreciate you doing the dishes. At the same time, it bothers me that after you do dishes, the floor is wet. I am worried that it will be a slipping hazard and damage the floor. I would really appreciate it if you could quickly wipe the wet spots on the ground after you're done doing dishes. Thank you for helping with the chores.

Emotional Regulation

TECHNIQUE #13: Self-Check-in Before and During Communication

Description: The patients check-in with themselves before and during the communication to see if this is a good time for it. If not, the patients can return to the conversation after cooling down.

Rationale: Builds on Chapter 2 Technique #3: Window of Tolerance. The patients need to be able to think and feel to convey the message. They need to regulate their emotions enough so the receiving party feels safe.

Note: Refer to the prior chapters' Stage 1 Skills for emotional regulation skills.

Script: Check in with yourself to see how you are feeling. Are you in your window of tolerance? What can you do to regulate your emotions and help yourself function optimally? Is this a good time for you to be having this conversation? If not, use an emotional regulation skill. Are you able to think before you say something (that you might regret later)?

If this is not a good time for you, or if you're not regulated, you need to communicate this.

Try saying I can't talk to you right now. I need to cool down.

Give the other person a timeline, so they know what to expect.

E.g., say "I will talk to you in ten minutes when I am feeling better."

TECHNIQUE #14: Planning Ahead

Description: The patients plan ahead for difficult conversations.

Rationale: Help the patients regulate their emotions before and after the communication so that they can be more successful and feel accomplished, controlling what they can control.

Script: Before you have a difficult conversation, I want you to plan what you will do so that you can regulate your emotions. In addition, plan what you will do after the conversation so that you can regulate yourself again.

Sample response: The patient says he'll do breathing exercises before the conversation. After the conversation, he'll go for a run.

TECHNIQUE #15: Writing as Communication

Description: Patients use writing to help with communication.

Rationale: Sometimes it is hard to figure out the right thing to say during the conversation. If the patients feel some things need to be communicated, but are not feeling confident that they can communicate them and stay calm, they can use writing as a medium to help.

Script: Try writing what you want to say in a letter and reading it to the other person. Then discuss it.

Communicate your wants, needs, thoughts, and feelings.

Ask for help. Read it over when you are calm, and edit or rewrite it. We will review it together before you read it to the other person.

TECHNIQUE #16: Acknowledging Emotions

Description: Acknowledge the other person's emotions.

Rationale: The other person also needs to feel heard and understood.

Script: I want you to name and acknowledge the other person's emotions. Acknowledging how the other person feels doesn't mean you agree with their action or behaviour.

Try, I can see that you are frustrated. It makes sense that you feel this way.

TECHNIQUE #17: De-escalation Skills

Description: Teach the patient de-escalation skills.

Rationale: People tend to mirror other people's emotions. They can use other people for emotional regulation.

Script: I want you to try and match the other person's tone, but pitch your voice a bit lower, and slowly bring it down.

Another strategy you can try is to say, I can't talk to you when you're yelling at me. I need you to lower your voice, so we can have a conversation.

You can also say, let's take a moment to cool down before we continue the conversation.

E.g., The patient says to the husband, let me give you a hug first. (The patient needs to know what the other person needs.)

Problem Solve and Negotiate

TECHNIQUE #18: Knowing Yourself

Description: The patient self-reflects on their goals, priorities, rights, etc.

Rationale: The patient needs to know what they want and how strongly they feel about it, so that they will know what to do.

Script: What do you need? What are you hoping to change? What specifically do you want?

What are your goals? What are your short-term goals? Long-term goals?

What are your priorities? Is it getting what you need? Is it the relationship (how others think and feel about the patient after the communication)? Is it self-respect (how you feel about yourself after the exchange)?

What do you hope for? What is typical and realistic? What is your bottom line?

What are your values, beliefs, rights, authorities?

Do you have the facts? Do the facts support your requests? Do you have the information you need to agree to something?

Are you able to fulfil the requests?

Do you feel this would be fair?

How much do you want this? What are you willing to do?

How will you feel about yourself?

What is the best timing for this? When is it good to say yes, to say no, to ask for something?

TECHNIQUE #19: Patients Gathering Information

Description: The patient considers information about the other person.

Rationale: Helps the patient see the other person's perspective.

Script: What information do you have about the other person? What information would be important to know?

What is the other person's intention? What are their priorities? What are their beliefs and values? What are their needs? What's their authority? What are their choices and alternatives? Do they understand what they are agreeing to? Are they able to fulfil your request?

TECHNIQUE #20: Reframing Unhelpful Thoughts

Description: Use Chapter 5: CBT to help reframe unhelpful thoughts and challenge myths.

Rationale: Unhelpful thoughts may be blocking the patient from having productive communication.

Script: What are some of your thoughts and beliefs about the communication that might be unhelpful?

E.g., "I don't deserve it," or "they don't deserve it," are unhelpful thoughts.

Is your fear of the consequences getting in the way? What is the worst thing that you can imagine happening?

E.g., The patient worries that she'll end up like her mother:

What are some myths?

E.g., I don't need other people.

What are more helpful thoughts?

Look forward to the future positives, rather than focusing on the past negatives.

E.g., Relationships are about give and take. Good communication is vital to a relationship. Conflicts present opportunities for change, new choices, relationship building, and improvement or growth.

TECHNIQUE #21: Exploring Strategies

Description: Explore different possibilities and choices.

Rationale: Some strategies may have worked previously or may apply in other settings, but don't work here.

Note: Childhood relationships and difficulties might come up. (See Chapter 8.) Consider prior relationships, including childhood relationships, and how they might affect the current relationship.

Script: What are some of the solutions you have thought about?

What strategies have you tried previously to get the support you need and to bring people closer to you?

How has this helped you previously? Do you think this is still effective? Why or why not?

Let's brainstorm strategies together, without judging them first. Then let's do pros and cons and come up with the best strategy.

Think about your interests and the other person's interests and how they may be aligned.

Look for win-win situations.

Try to save face.

Make it easy for people to say yes.

Think of the other person's perspective.

Make it appealing to both of you.

TECHNIQUE #22: Focusing on the Problem not the Person

Description: Focus on the problem, not the person.

Rationale: Focusing on the problem is more productive, and the other person doesn't feel hurt or attacked.

Script: People are not the same as the problem.

Don't blame others for the problem.

Don't attack the other person, e.g., don't say, "You're an idiot."

If the other person attacks, don't attack back; instead focus on the problem.

Think "good people make bad decisions," rather than "they are bad people."

Talk about finding solutions.

Open a discussion to generate solutions and brainstorm together.

Look for what's low value to you but high value to the other person for the give-and-take. Support with precedents and examples of how this has worked previously. Be reasonable.

TECHNIQUE #23: Positive Associations / Create Opportunistic Times

Description: Help the other person feel positively about the patient. Find an opportunistic time to interact with the other person.

Rationale: Improved relationships can help patients get what they want more easily.

Script: Find out what the other person likes.

E.g., The other person is most calm and happy after a meal. Make or get a lovely meal then negotiate after a meal. Find time to join the other person for meals or snacks to create positive associations. Think of timing and setting.

TECHNIQUE #24: Order of Requests

Description: Try arranging orders of request.

Rationale: Order of requests can help patients get what they want. Saying yes to one thing makes it easier to say yes to the next. After saying no to a big request, the person might feel bad and be open to a smaller request.

Script: Try:
- Starting with a small request and if the person agrees to it, try progressively increasing the request.
- Starting with a big request that you believe the other person will reject. Then try a smaller request and see if the other person will accept it.

TECHNIQUE #25: Researching Options

Description: Patients explore their options.

Rationale: Patients who know what their alternatives are can better decide and negotiate.

Script: Think of and research your options.

If the other person says no, what would you do? This will help you establish your bottom line and what you're willing to walk away from.

TECHNIQUE #26: Rewarding Good Behaviours

Description: Same concept as Chapter 5 Technique #14: Rewarding Desired Behaviour.

Rationale: Help the patient learn to influence others' behaviours.

Note: Teach the patient to try this consistently. If they are not consistent, the other person might learn to escalate.

Script: Give the other person praise when they're doing something you like or that is closer to the behaviour you want them to have.

E.g., Thank you for moving the dirty dishes to the counter beside the sink.

Plan rewarding experiences.

E.g., We've saved $1000 this month. Let's plan a quick weekend getaway.

TECHNIQUE #27: Therapist Role-Playing

Description: Considering all the above, the therapist can help plan the approach by using role-play with the patient.

Rationale: The therapist can help modify the approach and work together with the patient to address issues and suffering. The therapist teaches communications skills and helps refine them. The patient tries new behaviours and strategies.

Note: If it doesn't work, go back to brainstorming. Consider the potential consequences and reciprocity.

Script: Let's role-play it out so we can see how different options work and pick the best one.

TECHNIQUE #28: Ending the Relationship

Description: End relationships that are toxic.

Rationale: Sometimes the other person is unwilling to change. The patient would need to accept what cannot be changed. If this is unacceptable, then they need to know when to walk away and this includes terminating the relationship.

Script: Have you thought about ending the relationship? What does this say about you? How do you plan to do it? Who will support you?

Stage 2 Skills

TECHNIQUE #29: Grief

Description: Grief is a multidimensional response to loss. It has emotional, physical, cognitive, behavioural, social, and spiritual dimensions. It could stem from loss of health, job, relationship, person, pet, etc.

Help the patient grieve. Explore the positives and negatives. Explore complicated emotions, including ambivalence, guilt, and betrayal. Revisit the emotions and memories in a self-compassionate way. Grieve the loss, accept painful truths, and adapt to a new role.

Rationale: Sometimes the grieving is incomplete due to avoidance or lack of support. Help the patient connect with others so they can replace parts of what was lost with other relationships.

Note: Think about what was lost, such as innocence, childhood, hopes and dreams, identity (who they were), and trust. The patients may feel disillusioned.

Script: Tell me about the loss. What was happening then? Who was with you? What do you miss? What was the most difficult part of the experience? How did you feel about the other person?

What did you like and dislike about the other person? How did their actions affect your relationship?

What do you wish you could have said to the other person? What do you wish the other person could have said to you? What feels unfinished about this?

Looking back at what happened, how are you feeling? Who is supporting you through this?

Summary

Interpersonal relationships can be sources of conflict, but also sources of joy, fulfilment, and healing. IPT helps patients explore their relationships and self-reflect on changes and challenges. An effective communicator first gathers information by using active listening and tries to understand the other person's perspective. Using strategies such as taking turns to talk, "I" statements, and giving timely constructive feedback help the patient communicate their needs. For the communication to be effective, the patient needs to be emotionally regulated while delivering their messages and be mindful of how they are communicating, including non-verbally. While problem solving through conflicts and negotiating, it is important for the patient to consider their goals and values, focus on the problem rather than the person, and explore new solutions. The therapist can roleplay to help patients prepare for interpersonal interactions. Lastly, for an unhealthy relationship where the other person is unwilling to change or negotiate, the patient can end the relationship. Grieving helps the patient move on and find new healthy relationships.

CHAPTER 7:
Dialectical Behaviour Therapy (DBT) / Beyond the Classic CBT

This chapter contains more advanced techniques and combines skills from Chapters 1 to 6. It includes techniques from Dialectical Behaviour Therapy (DBT), Cognitive Processing Therapy (CPT), and Acceptance and Commitment Therapy (ACT).

In the late 1970s, DBT was created by Dr. Marsha Linehan to treat Borderline Personality Disorder (BPD), which is linked to childhood and developmental trauma. Developmental Trauma creates symptoms that overlap with BPD characteristics, such as dysregulation in mood, attention, behaviour, self, and relationships. (See Chapter 9 Knowledge #8: Developmental Trauma Disorder.) In addition to BPD, DBT is effective for the treatment of a wide range of disorders, including mood disorders, addictions, PTSD, eating disorders, self-harm, and suicidal behaviour. DBT teaches skills in mindfulness, emotional regulation, distress tolerance, and interpersonal effectiveness. This book covers mindfulness in Chapter 1, and interpersonal effectiveness in Chapter 6. Emotional regulation and distress tolerance are dispersed throughout the book in Stage 1 Skills. The DBT skills that combine techniques from previous chapters are covered here, including radical acceptance, STOP, and opposite action.

In the 1980s, Dr. Steven Hayes developed ACT and Dr. Patricia Resick et al. developed CPT. CPT uses CBT to challenge and process trauma related cognition and beliefs. (See Stage 2 Skills below for applying CBT to trauma.) ACT combines principles from CBT and mindfulness to help patients move towards their goals.

Trauma survivors can get stuck with powerful emotions that cause ongoing problems, such as anger, disgust, fear, guilt, shame, and mixed feelings. They can also be hampered by self-limiting or self-defeating beliefs and self-destructive behaviours. Using CBT to process the trauma narrative can help patients address trauma related emotions, beliefs, and behaviours and reintegrate the trauma.

Stage 1 Skills

TECHNIQUE #1: Radical Acceptance

Description: Patients fully accept what has happened and what cannot be changed as well as their feelings about the situation.

Rationale: Avoidance and non-acceptance make the situation worse. What's done cannot be undone.

Note: Radical acceptance doesn't imply that you approve of, agree with, forgive, or are glossing over an incident. Help patients tolerate their experiences, memories, emotions, and bodily sensations. Patients observe themselves and their experiences without judgment. They acknowledge their fears, insecurities, self-doubts, and feelings of helplessness and powerlessness.

Script: Sit with your palms facing up and a gentle smile. (See Chapter 1 Technique #14: Changing Body Position to Change Sensation.) Think about what you want to radically accept (e.g., losing your job). Observe your thoughts without judgment. (See Chapter 2 Technique #4: Judgments versus Facts.) When negative emotions arise, breathe through them. (See Chapter 1 Technique #1: Slow Outbreath.)

TECHNIQUE #2: STOP Skill

Description: A distress tolerance skill that brings in mindfulness.

Rationale: To tolerate intense emotions and not act rashly.

Script: When negative emotions are too intense, you STOP.

S: Stop.	Do not react.
T: Take a step back.	Breathe. Take a break. Think: "I am curious what thought will come to my mind next." This can stop racing thoughts.
O: Observe mindfully.	Observe your experience without judgment. Notice your thoughts and feelings. Distinguish the difference between the past and the present.
P: Proceed mindfully.	While being able to think and feel at the same time, find a balanced perspective. (See Chapter 2 Technique #6: Identifying States of Mind, Balanced Perspective.) What action do you want to take? Is this in line with your values and goals? Consider both short-term and long-term goals. (See Chapter 3 Technique #7: Values, and Technique #9: Setting Goals.) If you decide to take action, do so mindfully.

TECHNIQUE #3: Opposite Action

Description: Patients take the action that is opposite to their impulse.

Rationale: Doing the opposite can change how you feel and think about something.

Script: Think about an emotion that is preventing you from acting in alignment with your values or reaching your goals. To change that emotion, take the opposite action by changing your body posture, thoughts, perception, and action. Notice changes in your emotions and feelings about the situation.

	Current Emotion	Opposite Action
Body	Where in the body do you feel this?	Change your body posture. (See Chapter 1 Technique #14: Changing Body Position to Change Sensation.)
Thoughts	Observe your thoughts. Notice any hot thoughts. What do you believe about yourself in this situation? What do you believe about others?	Challenge hot thoughts. (See Chapter 5.)
Perception	What are you noticing?	Change the focus of your awareness.
Action	What action do you want to take?	Mindfully take the opposite action.

Stage 2 Skills

ABCs of CBT for Trauma (Build on Chapter 5 Skills)

Note: See Chapter 9 for information on psychological trauma.

Trauma alters **A**ffect (emotion), **B**ehaviour, and **C**ognition (beliefs and thoughts).

Patients who have been traumatized can have altered:

- Affect: difficulty identifying emotion; difficulty tolerating emotion; overwhelming fear, guilt, shame, and anger.
- Behaviour: avoidance, frequent safety-seeking and clinginess, overly controlling, and pathological coping,

self-soothing, and addictions. (See Chapter 9 Knowledge 10: Pathological Self-soothing / Addiction.)
- Cognition: distorted views based on generalizing trauma to other situations, "all or nothing" thinking.

Goals of using CBT for trauma:
- Affect: feel emotions. Tolerate emotions rather than feeling overwhelmed by negative emotions.
- Behaviour: remember, accept, and don't avoid the experience, minimize intrusiveness of the memories. (See Chapter 5 Techniques #19-22: Exposure Treatment.)
- Cognition: recognize helpful versus unhelpful thoughts and have more realistic and accurate thoughts.

Pre-treatment ABC Example

Affect	Behaviour	Cognition
Anxious, lonely.	Withdrawn.	The world is dangerous.

Post-treatment ABC Example

Affect	Behaviour	Cognition
Feeling confident, calm, and happy.	Maintains social connections and supports.	I survived. I did my best. It happened when I was a child and I didn't have control. There are parts of the world and people that are unsafe, but there are also good people out there. Now I have good social support and I am an independent adult.

Changing Trauma-Related Emotions

Assess whether the emotion is appropriate versus inappropriate or out of proportion with the situation. Appropriate emotions are in alignment with the patient's values and goals and reflect the present situation rather than the past.

Chapter 1 Technique #1: Slow Outbreath, and Chapter #7 Technique 2: STOP Skill can be applied to all of the following emotions.

TECHNIQUE #4: Anger

Description: Work with inappropriate anger.

Rationale: Anger allows people to take action to protect themselves from danger and defend their rights and boundaries, making them feel motivated and powerful. However, inappropriate anger can get in the way of relationships and create isolation. Uncontrolled anger may also lead to problematic behaviours. Anger may replace expressions of other emotions and become a way to avoid dealing with the underlying emotion. Help the patient be consistently assertive rather than have explosive anger, and to express anger in a healthy way. (See Chapter 6 Technique #8: "I" Statement.)

Script: How can you address inappropriate anger?

Opposite action	Anger	Opposite
Body	Clenched jaw and fists.	Relax jaw and fists.
Thoughts	It's unfair. That person is annoying.	Try to be compassionate. Imperfection is a part of being human. Wish the other person well. (See Chapter 3 Technique #6: Self-Compassion, and apply the same principles to the other person.)

Opposite action	Anger	Opposite
Perception	That person is getting in my way.	See Chapter 6 Technique #22: Focusing on the Problem not the Person.
Action	Attack and defend.	Befriend, be kind, forgive, or avoid. (See Chapter 3 Technique #20: Forgiving Others.)

TECHNIQUE #5: Disgust

Description: Work with inappropriate disgust.

Rationale: Disgust allows people to move away from health hazards (e.g., bodily fluids, poison), other people who are hurtful or violate their values, and unwanted sexual contact. However, inappropriate disgust can lead to obsessive compulsive cleaning, washing, and nausea or vomiting from trauma reminders. The fear of contamination can spread and generalize.

Script: How can you address inappropriate disgust?

Opposite action	Disgust	Opposite
Body	Nausea, vomiting, tense abdomen, and scrunched up face.	Relax face and abdomen.
Thoughts	I am contaminated or dirty.	See Chapter 4 Technique #5: Imagining Cleansing.

Opposite action	Disgust	Opposite
Perception	Perceive odour. Focus on body parts that are perceived as dirty.	Focus on the present moment. Distinguish the present from the past. (See Chapter 1 Technique #2: Orienting to the Present, and Technique #3: Engaging the Five Senses.) Focus on body parts that are clean or acceptable.
Action	Washing and cleaning. Avoiding healthy things that reminds the patient of the trauma, e.g., a patient who was sexually assaulted now fully avoids intimacy.	Do not clean or wash unless needed. (See Chapter 5 Exposure Treatment.) Eat mindfully. (See Chapter 1 Technique #4: One Mindful Thing, and apply it to eating.)

TECHNIQUE #6: Fear

Description: Technique to work with inappropriate fear.

Rationale: Fear motivates people to escape from danger. However, fear can limit people's exploration, experiences, and lives.

Script: How can you address inappropriate fear?

Opposite action	Fear	Opposite
Body	Heart palpitations, shallow breathing, chest tightness, raised shoulders, and hunched over.	Take a deep breath. Move shoulders down and back.

Opposite action	Fear	Opposite
Thoughts	How do I survive or escape? I am going to die.	Is the danger real? Check the facts. (See Chapter 5 Technique #7: Facts Supporting, Facts Against.) There's nothing to fear and I am safe.
Perception	Looking for danger.	Look for what signals safety.
Action	Run away, avoid, get help, or dissociate.	Face the situation. (See Chapter 5 Exposure Treatment Techniques #19-22.) Use grounding and mindfulness strategies. (See Chapter 1 Stage 1 Skills.)

TECHNIQUE #7: Guilt

Description: Technique to work with inappropriate guilt.

Rationale: Guilt motivates people to make atonement and act in alignment with their values. Sometimes traumatized patients try to make sense of what happened by blaming themselves. Guilt gives a sense of predictability to the world. People may need to admit that they are powerless to let go of the guilt.

Note: Guilt is about the behaviour: "I did something bad." Shame is about the self: "I am bad." There's no need to feel guilty about fantasies because they are not action. Some patients (e.g., child abuse survivors) have survivor's guilt and feel like they don't deserve to live. Therefore, congratulating someone for "surviving" may be triggering and make the patient feel guilty.

Script: How can you address inappropriate guilt?

Opposite action	Guilt	Opposite
Body	Hunched over and looking down.	Head up, shoulders back, and relax face.
Thoughts	I hate myself. I don't deserve this. It's my fault.	Consider who else is also responsible for the outcome. (See Chapter 5 Technique #9: Assigning Responsibility.) Think of things you are proud of. (See Chapter 3 Technique #12: Self-Esteem.) Think about what a friend would say. (See below for Technique #15: Role-playing Friend.)
Perception	Focus on criticism and weakness.	Look for positives. (See Chapter 3 Fostering Positive Experiences.)
Action	Submit, self-punish, apologize, and confess.	Face it. Treat yourself. Forgive yourself. (See Chapter 3 Technique #19: Self-Forgiveness.) Be proud. (See Chapter 3 Technique #12: Self-Esteem.) Let other people get to know you. (See Chapter 6, Technique #11: Practicing Self-Disclosures and Small Favours.)

TECHNIQUE #8: Shame and Self-Blame

Description: Technique to work with inappropriate shame.

Rationale: Shame and self-blame can give people a sense of self-awareness to maintain good relationships. Shame motivates them to change and improve the situation. Shame is relational. People feel shame because of their connection to others. Inappropriate shame makes people hide and disconnect from others and self. This can lead to chronic loneliness. Secrecy and judgment fuel shame, so doing the opposite reduces shame.

Note: Sometimes problematic behaviour used to cope with the painful feeling of shame worsens the shame, which in turn then worsens the behaviour. Don't judge it.

Script: How can you address inappropriate shame?

Opposite action	Shame	Opposite
Body	Curled up. Nausea.	Open up your chest, sit forward, and breathe in.
Thoughts	Self-critical thoughts: "I hate myself for what happened." "I should have done the right thing." "I should have been in control."	Self-compassion and self-love: "I'm not the same helpless person that I was."
Perception	Self-doubt.	Self-confidence. (See Chapter 3 Technique #12: Self-Esteem.)
Action	Submit or hide. Attack others or themselves.	Set healthy boundaries. See opposite action for Chapter 7 Technique #7: Guilt. Reveal the secret. (See Chapter 8 Technique #14: Secrecy and Truth Telling.)

What would you do if you didn't have that shame? (See below for Technique #20: Future Orientation and Focusing on Positives.) Try reframing the situation. E.g., instead of saying, "I'm sorry I'm late," reframe it as, "Thank you for waiting." This turns shame into gratitude. (See Chapter 3 Technique #4: Reframing.)

TECHNIQUE #9: Mixed Emotions

Description: Technique to work with mixed emotions.

Rationale: It's natural to have mixed emotions. Emotions motivate people to take action. Conflicting emotions signal opposite actions. When people have intense mixed emotions, they create intense inner tension and confusion.

Note: Mixed up feelings: take pleasure in pain, love hate, trust what's dangerous, etc.

Script: How can you address intense mixed emotions?

Try STOP skill:

S: Stop.

T: Take a step back. Breathe.

O: Observe your thoughts and emotions. Name the emotions that come up.

P: Proceed mindfully after balancing the perspectives.

(See Techniques #4-8 to address the individual emotions.)

(See Chapter 2 Technique #6: Identifying States of Mind, Balanced Perspective, and Chapter 5 Technique #16: Putting it Together.)

Changing Trauma-Related Beliefs

TECHNIQUE #10: Identifying Trauma-Related Beliefs

Description: Identifying hot thoughts that are related to the trauma.

Rationale: Help patients recognize the hot thoughts that are related to their trauma. Old beliefs may no longer serve the patient well. The patient needs to create more balanced and helpful cognitive beliefs. Sometimes patients are stuck in a self-fulfilling prophecy and need to reset expectations in order to have more functional and healthier lives.

Script: Here is a list of hot thoughts that are trauma-related. Let's review them together. Let me know which ones you identify with.

Trauma affects beliefs about:

1) Self

2) Relationships and other people

3) World

Regarding:

1) Control:
- Agency and power
- Inhibition
- Standards
- Boundaries

2) Self-esteem / Self-definition / Self-care

3) Safety / Trust

4) Disconnection

Self
- Control:
    - It's all my fault.
    - I deserved to be punished.
    - I'm inadequate or a failure. I won't ever measure up to others. I will never survive on my own.
    - If I don't control my emotions, they will control me and I will lose control of my actions.
    - I need to be perfect. I shouldn't make mistakes. I beat myself up for my mistakes.
    - I am impulsive and cannot control my behaviour.
    - I'm incapable. I don't have the concentration to complete tasks.
- Self-esteem / Self-definition / Self-care:
    - I am broken / damaged / abnormal.
    - I'm crazy.
    - I am unintelligent.
    - I am unattractive.
    - I'm unworthy. I don't deserve it.
    - I ignore my needs.
    - I constantly feel "not good enough."
- Safety / Trust:
    - I am going to die young (foreshortened future).
    - I worry a lot about my health even when there's no medical reason to.
    - I can't trust myself / my judgments / decisions / thoughts / feelings / intuition.
- Disconnection:
    - I don't belong. I don't need anyone.
    - I am unlovable. I am invisible.

Relationships
- Control:
    - I'm special and standard rules shouldn't apply to me.
    - I don't accept other people saying "no" to me.
    - I need lots of praise and constant reassurance.
    - I set low expectations so I won't be disappointed.
    - I can't say no. I am a people pleaser. I let other people make decisions for me.
    - I hold grudges and don't accept excuses from others.
    - I don't express how I feel to other people.
- Self-esteem / Self-definition / Self-care:
    - Others don't care about me.
    - Others don't respect me.
    - Others don't treat me fairly.
    - I have difficulty having separate identities and setting boundaries with people (partner, parents, etc.)
    - I sacrifice myself for people whom I love and care about. I don't have time to take care of myself. I'm the one caring for others around me.
- Safety / Trust:
    - Others cannot be trusted or relied upon.
    - I cannot depend on others for support.
    - Other people are unpredictable / unreliable.
    - Others will take advantage of me / abuse or exploit me.
    - Others only act nice towards me because they want something from me.
    - I should try to hurt the other person first if I think they're trying to hurt me.

- I expect relationships to end and sometimes will pre-emptively drive people away.
- I like to "test" other people.
* Disconnection:
- Others will abandon or leave me. People will leave me if they know who I am or if I express myself.
- No one understands me. I need to hide my true self from others.
- No one would miss me if I'm gone.
- I am attracted to people who reject me.

World

* Control:
    - The world is unpredictable. The world is what it is and I have no control.
    - The world is hopeless and bleak.
* Self-esteem / Self-definition / Self-care:
    - I just take up space in this world.
* Safety / Trust:
    - The world is dangerous.
* Disconnection:
    - I am alone in this world.

Variation A: Meaning of Traumatic Events

Description: Explore the meaning of traumatic events.

Rationale: Trauma can strengthen prior negative beliefs.

Script: How have these events affected your belief about yourself, others, and the world?

What did the experience say about you?

Of the bad things that happened, what did you think about the most or hate thinking about the most?

How did you feel about sharing it?

TECHNIQUE #11: Hot Thoughts in Context of Trauma

Description: Identifying trauma-related hot thoughts.

Rationale: Once the patient can identify the hot thoughts, they can change them.

Script: Here is a list of trauma related hot thoughts and examples. Let's review them together. I want you to write down your hot thoughts and bring them to our next clinic.

- All or Nothing Thinking: Since my boyfriend can't be there for me during my exam preparation, he can never be there for me.
- Shoulds: I should have done better.
- Jumping to Conclusions: When bad things happen, it is my fault.
- Mental Filter: I discount my accomplishments and only focus on failures. This makes me feel "not good enough."
- Labelling: I am worthless.
- Double Standard: Rules apply to others but not to me.
- Magnification / Catastrophizing / Blowing Things Out of Proportion: Because I was sexually assaulted, no man would ever want me.
- Emotional Reasoning: I feel guilty and therefore I am.
- Blaming: My parents screwed me up.
- Over-Generalizing: All people in power exploit those they oversee.
- Magical Thinking: If I can make the traumatic event unhappen, my life would be perfect.

TECHNIQUE #12: CBT Recording for Trauma

Description: Doing CBT recording for trauma-related hot thoughts.

Rationale: Recording them brings awareness.

Script:

Situation	Thoughts	Emotions and Intensity
Parents placed responsibility on the patient as a child to care for siblings and offered no support.	I'm incompetent. I should have done a better job. I am responsible. I am worthless.	Shame: 90. Guilt: 90.

Bodily Sensation	Behaviour
Feels butterflies in the stomach, wants to hide. Feels suffocated.	Avoids thinking about this. Drinks alcohol to avoid feeling.

TECHNIQUE #13: Challenging Trauma-Related Beliefs

Description: Challenge the thoughts. (Continue from the above Technique #12.)

Rationale: To create more balanced thoughts.

Script:

Facts Supporting	Facts Against
My brother is homeless and struggles with addiction.	My sister has a stable job. I made sure they had food. I cooked meals when I was nine years old.

TECHNIQUE #14: Assigning Responsibility to Trauma

Description: Applying Chapter 5 Technique #9: Assigning Responsibility to trauma.

Rationale: Help reduce self-blame.

Script: Who else was responsible for taking care of your siblings? Who else is responsible for how they turned out?

E.g., Parents, teachers, other family members, siblings, etc.

TECHNIQUE #15: Role-Playing Friend

Description: Patient role-playing a friend.

Rationale: Help patients have more self-compassion and gain perspective.

Script: I am going to role-play you. I want you to role-play your friend.

Sample response: Therapist: I did a terrible job raising my siblings. I am worthless.

Patient: You were just a child. Your parents were responsible for looking after them. You did your best.

Variation A: Role-play Giving Advice to Old Self

Description: The therapist role-plays the patient in the past.

Rationale: Give patients the power to give advice. They can see the difference between now and then.

Script: What advice would you give your old self? Imagine your adult self walking into the scene. I'll role-play you.

Sample response: Patient: You have terrible parents. You're doing your best. You'll grow up one day and this will all be easier.

TECHNIQUE #16: Going into Trauma Details

Description: Use the five senses to go into the patient's trauma.

Rationale: Do exposure therapy by going into the details of the traumatic memory. Patients tend to only tell the parts of the story that they can tolerate. There's frequently more unprocessed content that could be accessed by asking questions about the five senses.

Caveat: This can be very triggering. Go back and forth between using emotional regulation skills and getting details of the trauma. Combine this with Stage 1 Skills, Chapter 3 Technique #6: Self-Compassion, and Chapter 4 Technique #16: Adding Imaginary Elements. (See Chapter 9 Psychological Trauma.)

Script: Describe the worst part of the memory in detail.

What was happening? How old were you? Where were you? What were you doing? Who was there? What did you see, hear, feel, smell, and taste?

TECHNIQUE #17: Narrative Exposure

Description: Practice writing traumatic events in detail.

Rationale: Given that memory is reconstructed, narrating the trauma helps to integrate the traumatic memory into general memory. During the trauma, people freeze and later are unable to talk about the experience. Help patients to tolerate the memory and create a coherent narrative. By facing the negative experiences, sometimes the patient is also able to remember the positive experiences. When patients find language to convey their inner experience, they can feel more connected and less lonely. Language can also serve as a substitute for action. Putting the traumatic memory into words can help prevent re-enactments. (See Chapter 8 Knowledge #3: Traumatic Re-enactment.)

Note: Start with simple questions to see if the patient can tolerate them before getting into full details of the trauma. Listen for missing details / events. Get the original story before challenging the thoughts. Write it down. Pace the story and slow down, especially to help with emotional regulation. This builds on Chapter 3 Technique #18: Rewriting Your Story and Reframing.

Script: What is abuse?

Why do you think it happened?

What does that say about you?

Let's create a timeline of your life.

What was going on in your life before the traumatic event?

What was the first, worst, and most recent event that happened?

(Optional: put rocks on the negative events and petals on the positive events.)

Variation A: Table of Contents

Description: Creating a table of contents first, then filling out the details.

Script: Let's create a table of contents. It will have easier sections and ones with trauma. Once we have created the table of contents, we will fill out the details. (Probe by saying, "Tell me more.") Which section do you want to work on?

Variation B: Journaling about Traumatic Events

Description: Patients write their stories on their own.

Rationale: This allows patients to go in-depth and explore themselves without fearing judgment from others.

Note: This builds on Chapter 2 Technique #12: Journaling. As before, the therapist does not need to know the details. Check-in on how this is working for them and invite the patients to share only if they want to.

Script: I want you to write your story in a journal. You do not need to share it with me, but I am here for you if there's anything you would like to share. Let me know how that goes.

TECHNIQUE #18: Staying Grounded while Processing Traumatic Memory

Description: Tips to help the patient explore the traumatic memory, yet stay grounded in the present.

Rationale: Exposing patients to their traumatic content can be overwhelming. The intent is not for the patient to relive the experience. Instead, help the patient explore the memory in a way that is self-compassionate and tolerable emotionally, while staying in the present.

Script: It is important that you stay with me rather than relive the traumatic experience. Stay with me. On a scale of one to ten, how present are you?

(If not ten, what can we do to help you come back to the present and be with me? Let's do an emotional regulation exercise. Of all the skills you've learned, which one would you like to use? Use a Stage 1 Skill.)

Stay with the memory and the present experience if you can tolerate them. Remember that natural emotions come and go. (See Chapter 2 Technique #13: Observing Emotions.)

TECHNIQUE #19: Challenging the Meaning of Traumatic Events

Description: Challenge the meaning of the traumatic events.

Rationale: Sometimes the story becomes an alibi. Instead of tuning into emotions, the recital of misery leads to more misery. Visiting the trauma needs to be done mindfully, so the patient can reconnect with themselves and re-think about it compassionately. The trauma is part of their identity rather than the entire identity.

Note: Build on Technique #10: Identifying Trauma-related Beliefs.

Script: How did you feel about the traumatic experience? What does that say about you? Is this interpretation reasonable given the context or far from reality?

Sample response: Patient: It tells me that I'm stupid.

Therapist Responses using Different Techniques:
- You feel you are not smart. What are facts supporting and facts against this? (Process trauma using CBT.)
- The self-critical part of you says you're not smart. What does that do for you? Talk with that part of you and address the conflict. (See Chapter 5 Technique #17: Ambivalence / Working with Parts.)
- Ideal parents believe you are smart. (See Chapter 4 Technique #9: Variation A: Imagining Ideal Parents.)

TECHNIQUE #20: Birthday Speech

Description: Pretend that a friend is giving a birthday speech about the patient's life.

Rationale: Seeing the situation from a different perspective can reduce distress.

Script: Imagine that your friend is giving a birthday speech about your life at your party. What would you like your friend to say? What details would you focus on? What are you most proud of? What would you want to omit? Could you rephrase the things you want to omit?

Variation A: Talk Show Host

Description: The therapist pretends to be a talk show host interviewing the patient "expert."

Rationale: For use with children. View the situation from the position of "expert" rather than "victim."

Script: Therapist: Welcome to our talk show. Today, we are interviewing an expert with experience in dog bites. What did you learn from your dog bite experience?

Patient: You have to be careful around dogs.

Therapist: How do you know if a dog is going to bite or not?

Patient: You don't until you get to know the dog.

Therapist: How do you get to know a dog?

Patient: You can talk to the owner. You can approach the dog carefully. If the dog is growling, don't keep approaching.

TECHNIQUE #21: Future Orientation and Focusing on Positives

Description: Looking into the future with hope.

Rationale: Help patients realize that the trauma was in the past. Help them look forward to the future with hope, because there is more to their life than the trauma. Most of CBT is challenging negatives, but it is just as important to build on positives and they can be combined. Sometimes when patients can process the bad things they can also recall the good things about a specific situation or person.

Note: Don't force the silver lining as it can be invalidating. (See Chapter 3 Technique #13: Fostering Hope and Optimism.)

Script: The trauma was in the past. How is the past different from your present situation?

What would you tell others in your previous situation?

Sample response: Patient: I'm an independent adult. I managed to protect my own children from being abused. I would tell others to listen to what their children have to say.

Changing Trauma-Related Behaviour

TECHNIQUE #22: Mindfulness of Craving

Description: Bringing mindful awareness to the sensation of craving.

Rationale: Wanting creates stress and pain. Paying attention to it can decrease the craving. Help patients train their ability to focus on long-term goals rather than short-term gain.

Script: Notice what the experience of wanting feels like. Try to distract yourself for ten minutes. Try to substitute something else.

E.g., Direct your attention to the sensation of craving food. Notice what you are craving. Try to distract yourself for ten minutes. Try having something healthy such as celery. Notice how your desire for food decreases as you mindfully eat.

E.g., Direct your attention to the sensation of craving cigarettes. Try to distract yourself for ten minutes. Try mindfully substituting some sugarless lozenges. Notice how your desire for a cigarette changes when you bring mindfulness to it.

TECHNIQUE #23: ACT

Description: Use ACT.

Rationale: Help patients move towards their goals.

Script:

1) Be present / mindful.

2) Radical acceptance (See Technique #1.)

3) Use cognitive techniques: Observe your thoughts and change unhelpful thoughts to reduce emotional distress. E.g., Sing your thoughts or change them to a kinder tone. (See Chapter 5 CBT.)

4) "Self as context:" People are more than the sum of their experiences, thoughts, and feelings.

5) Evaluate your values and both short-term and long-term goals. (See Chapter 3 Technique #7: Values, and Technique #9: Setting Goals.)

6) Take action mindfully.

Summary

Combining CBT with other therapies creates powerful techniques that can be used to treat a wide range of disorders. When using narrative exposure, it is important for the patient to tolerate their emotions and stay grounded in the present. Help patients explore their traumatic memory in a self-compassionate way instead of reliving the experience. By using CBT to process past trauma, patients can move from intense and intolerable negative emotions to tolerable emotions that more accurately reflect the present situation. This helps patients have more balanced and realistic thoughts. Moreover, it reduces addictive behaviours, increases helpful behaviours, and moves patients towards their goals. Once patients can process bad experiences, they can better recall good experiences and integrate new experiences. Using CBT to process trauma helps patients realize the trauma is over and now they can look forward to the future with optimism.

Part II: Applications

CHAPTER 8:
Attachment and the Therapeutic Relationship

In the 1900s, Dr. John Bowlby developed Attachment Theory. He believed attachment difficulty between the infant and primary caregiver could lead to detrimental long-term consequences, including issues with cognition, mood, and relationships. He also believed that attachment difficulty can be transmitted to the next generation. In the 1970s, Dr. Mary Ainsworth did the "strange situation" experiment to observe and categorize types of infant attachments.

The therapist is a caregiver and therefore can activate the patient's attachment system and previous relationship patterns. Attachment is also activated when patients feel threatened or fearful (e.g., when a patient is unwell). The attachment to the therapist can create a healing environment for the patient to explore and understand themselves, but also has the potential to create challenges. This relationship between the therapist and the patient is the key component for moving the patient towards recovery and is more important than what specific technique you choose to practice.

This chapter discusses types of attachment and the challenges caused by different insecure attachment types. It introduces techniques to treat attachment disorders and move patients from insecure to secure attachments. When traumatized patients engage in traumatic re-enactment with a therapist, strategies are needed to address the situation. This chapter illustrates ways to structure and provide trauma-informed therapy and repair the therapeutic relationship.

KNOWLEDGE #1: Attachments

#1a: Definition and Types

Attachment is how one person connects with another. An infant develops bonds to its parents. They have inborn behaviour to help develop closeness with caregivers. Attachment style and patterns are also shaped by experiences. A child takes cues from parents. Caregivers are usually the source of security for the child, but this isn't always the case.

Attachment styles are secure versus insecure. Insecure attachment styles are sometimes labelled attachment disorders.

Secure Attachment
- Healthy sense of self and mentalizing skills
- Able to use others for emotional support and emotional regulation
- Comfortable with closeness and being alone
- Able to explore
- Has a flexible balance between reliance on self versus others and balance between expressing versus suppressing display of emotions

Insecure Attachment

The three types of insecure attachments are anxious / preoccupied, dismissing / avoidant, and disorganized.

1) Anxious / Preoccupied
- Fear of being alone and abandonment
- Rejection sensitivity and frequently seeking approval
- Compulsive caretaking of others
- Jealousy

2) Dismissing / Avoidant
- Dismissing behaviour
- Mistrusts others
- Fear of closeness and difficulty getting close to others
- Downplays emotions
- False sense of self-sufficiency

3) Disorganized
- Features of both anxious / preoccupied and dismissing / avoidant attachments
- Emotional dysregulation, poor mentalizing ability
- Splitting between different states of mind, extremes between controlling and submissive
- Unstable in relationships
- Difficulty with exploring and self-agency

#1b: Etiology

Secure Attachment

Parents are attuned and meet the child's psychological and physical needs consistently enough.

Insecure Attachments

1) Anxious / Preoccupied: Parents discourage exploring behaviour and want the child to be attached to them. Parents are mis-attuned or unresponsive. There is a role reversal where the parents want the child to be attuned to them and help the parents regulate their emotions. Parents are multitasking and dragging the child into what they're doing.

2) Dismissing / Avoidant: Parents are rejecting when a child seeks out physical and emotional closeness. Parents mis-attune to a child's negative emotions and instead encourage the child to be

independent and autonomous. Parents are controlling and directly play for the child, rather than play with the child collaboratively.

3) Disorganized: Parents activate defence responses / systems (such as fight / flight) and attachment system, which creates a dilemma because they are contradicting systems, i.e., the source of attachment is also a source of fear. (See Chapter 9 Knowledge #15: Defence Responses.)

#1c: Distinguishing Types of Attachment

Adult Attachment Interview (AAI): This is an interview that asks the patients to describe their immediate family and their relationship with their parents when they were young children. Use five adjectives to describe the relationship with their mother / father and provide evidence to support each.

Note: This book only provides a brief description of the AAI, so some therapists may choose to receive additional training in this.

Secure Attachment
- Able to provide a coherent story and able to mentalize
- Able to emotionally regulate, and able to think and feel at the same time
- Reflects on the experience in a self-compassionate way
- The details provided make sense and support the chosen adjectives

Insecure Attachments

1) Anxious / Preoccupied
- Tells long stories with difficulty staying focused. The story contains contradictions.
- Preoccupied with past relationships
- Uses jargon or has difficulty finding words

- Anger towards the caregiver
- Role reversals

2) Dismissing / Avoidant
- Short story with lack of emotion and details
- Dismisses the experience or has an idealized view of it despite the neglect
- Suppresses the distress
- Talks about social norms / roles instead of actual self-reflections. There is a lack of mentalizing.

3) Disorganized
- Elements of both anxious / preoccupied and dismissing / avoidant
- Both the attachment system and the defence responses are activated and they create a dilemma
- Disorganized story and disconnected ideas including intrusive or odd thoughts
- Sometimes prolonged silence and sometimes tangential and drawn out
- Missing details about trauma and loss
- The patient is inflexible and dysregulated
- Difficulty mentalizing
- "Borderline"

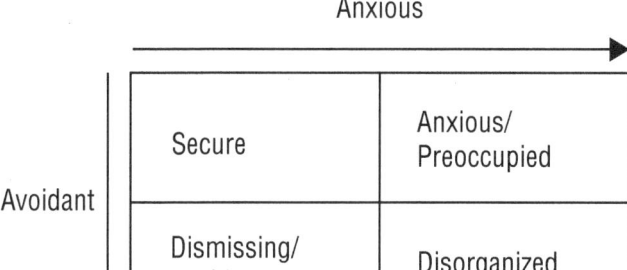

Figure 4: Types of Attachments

#1d: Approach to Insecure Attachments

1) <u>Anxious / Preoccupied</u>
    - Main thing to activate: Exploration
    - Therapist to:
        - Be consistent and predictable.
        - Be present, attuned, and genuine.
        - Be a calm presence
    - Affect: Teach skills to reduce anxiety.
    - Relationship / Communication:
        - Teach assertiveness.
        - Teach patients not to use jargon.
        - Teach turn-taking during the conversation.
    - Self:
        - Encourage exploration.
        - Self-agency.
        - Self-esteem. (See Chapter 3 Technique #12: Self-Esteem.)

2) Dismissing / Avoidant
- Main thing to activate:
    - Attachment.
    - Some patients feel shame when they feel attachment needs. Validate that it's normal to want relationships / connections.
- Therapist to:
    - Be attuned to emotions, including negative ones.
    - Respect interpersonal distance / independence.
    - Schedule appointments, rather than as needed appointments.
- Affect:
    - Emphasize feelings and teach that emotions can help the patient get closer to people and not more distant.
    - Allow patients to grieve (the loss of childhood and how little they got from their parents).
- Relationship / Communication:
    - Work on collaborating with the therapist.
    - Find common ground and common goals.
    - Teach non-verbal skills, e.g., making eye contact.
    - Patients are slow to warm up (takes time to reactivate attachment system), but once they get started they become faithful.
- Self: Be permissive and let patients explore (including exploring within themselves, their feelings, their motives behind behaviours, etc.)

3) Disorganized
- Main thing to activate:
    - Exploration and attachment.
    - Address fear of attachment.

- - Use strategies from both Anxious / Preoccupied and Dismissing / Avoidant.
- Therapist to:
  - Be aware of changes in states of mind.
  - Set appropriate boundaries.
- Affect:
  - Allow patients to communicate emotions and validate their feelings. (See Chapter 2 Technique #1: Teaching Language for Emotions.)
  - Help patients be present / grounded.
- Relationship / Communication: Use strategies from both Anxious / Preoccupied, and Dismissing / Avoidant.
- Self:
  - Instil hope.
  - Teach metacognitive skills.

KNOWLEDGE #2: Understanding "Challenging Patients" Through Attachment and Countertransference

Survivors of interpersonal trauma tend to have difficulty trusting and feeling safe with others and may fear the attachment to the therapist. Their defence response may turn on when the therapist gets close. (See Knowledge #15: Defence Response.) Conversely, their attachment system may turn on when the therapist tries to get further away. This paradoxical behaviour can be challenging for the therapist.

Transference: Patients redirect their feelings about someone else onto the therapist.

Countertransference: The therapist redirects their feelings about someone else onto the patient. This can occur in response to transference. It can be problematic when it brings up the therapist's own unresolved issues.

"Challenging" patients stir up strong negative feelings in the caregiver, such as hate, anger, resentment, hopelessness, helplessness, and anxious feelings. Most of these patients have insecure attachment styles. Sometimes the therapist finds the patient "challenging" because they are stuck in a traumatic re-enactment (see below.)

KNOWLEDGE #3: Traumatic Re-enactment

Traumatic re-enactment can happen more readily in patients with early age trauma. Children first develop imitative memory, then fully develop narrative memory around age four. Hence, in early age trauma, the patient has predominantly behavioural and not narrative memory for the trauma. Since procedural memory leads to automatic behaviour, the patient then acts out the trauma. Thinking creates choices and can help stop the automatic behaviour.

For example, a three-year-old child was abused and choked by an adult. When playing with a doll, the child chokes the doll and ties elastic bands around the doll's neck. However, the child is unable to tell the story.

Many survivors of childhood trauma have different parts / self-states that play different roles. Working through these parts helps reduce the risk of re-enactment. The re-enactment can occur within the patient (e.g., self-critical voice) or between the patient and another person, such as the therapist.

Self-states

- Victim: Feels helpless. Doesn't take responsibility and blames others. Dependent on others.
- Abuser: Feels entitled and powerful. Aggressive, abusive, and vengeful. Hurts others or oneself.
- Saviour: Feels responsible for saving others and solving their problems, even at personal expense.
- Bystander: Fails to protect or intervene when needed.

Treatments
- Victim: Empower them to take responsibility and action.
- Abuser: Empathize, be able to feel and be vulnerable, and assertive rather than aggressive.
- Saviour: Observe and think before jumping in to help.
- Bystander: Accept that their neglect can cause harm.

When the traumatic re-enactment is between different parts of self, address this by using Chapter 5 Technique #17: Ambivalence / Working with Parts.

KNOWLEDGE #4: Limiting Therapist Self-Disclosure

Therapist self-disclosure may distract from the therapy. The therapist may be trying to solve their own unmet needs rather than focusing on the patient. This is a reversal of the therapeutic relationship (patient caring for therapist). The patient may feel the therapist is unable to handle their trauma. Disclose only what is needed to repair the relationship.

KNOWLEDGE #5: Therapist Stance for Trauma-Informed Care

Being trauma-informed is a stance that the therapist takes.

Note: This is a universal approach and doesn't just become relevant when the therapist obtains a trauma history. This increases the chance of integrating and recovering from trauma.

Components of trauma informed care (the twelve Cs):
- Connection: One of the most important is for the therapist to be present and attuned: aware of affect, non-verbal communication, and what's not said. (See Chapter 2 Technique #8: Therapist Attunement for Awareness, and Chapter 8 Technique #4: Connection.)

- Communicate clearly: Answer questions, explain the process, set expectations, and explain the limits of confidentiality. Use language and deliver content at the level appropriate for the patient, and avoid jargon. Establish rules of communication including turn-taking and responsiveness. Be genuine and truthful in the communication. (See Chapter 8 Technique #2: Setting Expectations, and #3: Sample Contract.)
- Collaborate: Find common ground, shared goals, and work together. (See Chapter 8 Technique #5: Priorities and Align Goal / Getting Buy-in.)
- Consistent: Uphold boundaries, be reliable, predictable, and schedule appointments. (See Chapter 8 Technique #7: Maintaining Boundaries.)
- Calm: Create a safe environment and provide containment. (See Chapter 8 Technique #8: Safety, and #9: Slowing Down the Process.)
- Choice: Empower the patient (See Chapter 8 Technique #10: Choice.)
- Curious: Come from a position of not knowing. (See Chapter 2 Technique #10: Curiosity and "I Wonder" Statements, and Chapter 8 Technique #11: Curious.)
- Compassionate: Be empathic, supportive, warm, and give appropriate validation. (See Chapter 8 Technique #12: Validation, and #13: Balance Between Validation and Challenge.)
- Create trust: Help with truth telling. (See Chapter 8 Technique #14: Secrecy and Truth Telling.)
- Create hope. (See Chapter 7 Technique #21: Future Orientation and Focusing on Positives.)
- Coping: Build resilience and use the patient's strengths. (See Chapter 3.)
- Cultural competence. (See Chapter 6.)

Structure Therapy

TECHNIQUE #1: Identifying Patient Baseline

Description: Take a social history.

Rationale: Taking a social history helps to build rapport and gives the therapist a sense of the patient's baseline. The techniques covered in this book work for people with cognitive impairment up to mild dementia. A social history helps the therapist get a sense of the patient's cognitive ability and make treatment decisions. Can the patient tell a story that doesn't have traumatic events? Sometimes when the patient tells a traumatic story, they become more disorganized and have difficulty.

Note: If the patient cannot tell a therapist key information, such as what their job was or what kind of education they had, they may be too cognitively impaired for the techniques in this book.

Script: I want to chat with you to get to know you better.

Can you start by telling me your name and age?

Where do you live?

Where were you born? Where did you grow up?

What's your first language?

What kind of education did you have?

What do you do for a living? (Or what did you do for a living? When did you retire?)

TECHNIQUE #2: Setting Expectations

Description: Be transparent and set the expectations regarding therapy, so the patient knows what to anticipate. Explain that therapists are humans and might not get it right, so patient feedback is important to guide treatment. The patient is expected to get better by moving towards the agreed upon goals and not regress.

Rationale: Setting the expectation helps establish predictability. Being consistent and predictable is calming. This can help the patient get out of survival mode so that they can begin to process information. Wording therapy as trial and error sets up expectations of two-way communication between patient and therapist. Let patients know that their voices are important and that they need to be heard.

Note: Make extending therapy contingent on the patient demonstrating an improvement so the therapist is rewarding good behaviour (instead of rewarding patients for staying ill).

Script: I do __ (e.g., weekly) therapy and the sessions are __ (e.g., twenty minutes long) and will go on for __ (number of weeks). (I may extend the therapy if I believe it is needed AND that you have demonstrated that you are getting better.) In therapy, we will try different techniques. Just because a technique works for most people, it doesn't mean it would necessarily be right for you. A large part of therapy will be trial and error, so your feedback is very important. It will help guide our work together. If something is not working for you or doesn't feel right, please let me know right away. My job is to help you get better and I have the best of intentions. At the same time, I won't necessarily get it right, so I need your help and your feedback. I expect people to get better during therapy. There may be some ups and downs depending on the day, but I expect the overall trajectory to be headed towards getting better and going towards our target goals.

TECHNIQUE #3: Sample Contract

Description: Creating a written contract between the therapist and the patient.

Rationale: The therapist has something to fall back on if the patient violates boundaries or engages in therapy-disrupting behaviours.

Script:

I, _____, agree to the following rules regarding therapy:

I will attend and participate in therapy. I will stay committed and collaborate in therapy.

I will cancel my appointment with at least a twenty-four-hour notice if I cannot attend therapy.

I will do my best to complete the homework.

I will work on stopping self-destructive behaviour, including addictive behaviours such as substance abuse, self-harm, and out-of-control eating.

I will not attempt suicide during treatment. I will seek immediate help if I am in crisis or have difficulty keeping myself safe.

I will not come to therapy under the influence of substances.

I will not behave violently or use abusive language.

I will notify my therapist about any other therapy or treatment that I am receiving.

I understand that my therapist works in a team and confidentiality is maintained within the team.

I understand that everything I say is kept confidential with some limits to confidentiality.

Limits to confidentiality include:
- If I am going to harm myself or someone else.
- If I am going to harm or have harmed a child or a senior in an institution.
- If the court requests the information for a legal case.
- If I request my information to be shared with a third party. I will sign a consent form for the release of confidential information to the indicated third party.

_____   _____
Signature of Patient   Date

TECHNIQUE #4: Connection

Description: Build connection with the patient.

Rationale: Doing Stage 1 Skills together can help foster the relationship and aid the therapist co-regulate with the patient. It aids with emotional connection during therapy as it's happening and can help the therapist be more aware of the patient's internal process. (See Knowledge #1: Relationship First.)

Script: Let's do the exercises together.

You're not alone. I'm here with you.

Let's talk about the experience. How does that make you feel? (Doing the exercise together helps the therapist relate better to the patient.)

TECHNIQUE #5: Priorities and Aligning Goals / Getting Buy-in

Description: Explore the patient's goals, wishes, and motivation. Explain what therapy will help them do.

Rationale: Part of the therapeutic alliance involves aligning the goals. Meet the patient where they are. Also, build on the patient's strengths and instil hope. The collaboration builds the connection.

Script: What made you seek treatment now? Why specifically now? What bothers you the most? What are you hoping to achieve? What do you think might help you achieve these goals?

E.g., The patient wants a better relationship with his family. The therapist identifies emotional regulation as a goal, but the patient did not list this.

Sample Response: Yes, we will work towards helping you have a better relationship with your family. I am also hearing that your emotions and anger are affecting your relationship. I feel that it is important for us to work on your ability to regulate your emotions, so you can be more successful in your relationships. How does this sound?

TECHNIQUE #6: Therapy-Disrupting Behaviour

Description: Recognize and address therapy-disrupting behaviour early.

Rationale: This reinforces the expectations. The therapist and patient can explore and problem-solve through this together.

Script: I notice that ____ (e.g., you are coming late to our sessions.) This is affecting the therapy.

What do you think is causing this behaviour?

What could you do to address this?

Examples of therapy-disrupting behaviours:

- Destabilizing between treatments: Making extra demands or having frequent crises such as going to Emergency or extra calls to the therapist. Regression in function, violating therapist's privacy, and self-destructive behaviours.
  - E.g., Regression: patient fears getting hurt / abandonment and fears having new expectations when they are better.
- Not following the treatment plan: Missing appointments with therapist and other practitioners, not taking medication, incomplete homework, and refusing to let the therapist speak with others in the circle of care.
- Disrupting therapy sessions: Coming intoxicated or late, being abusive or inappropriate towards the therapist, refusing to end the session, lying, long silences, refusing to talk about certain topics, and dominating the session.

Make extending therapy contingent on the patient demonstrating an improvement. (See Technique #2: Setting Expectations.) List the pros and cons of getting better. (See Chapter 2 Technique #11: Pros and Cons.) Empower patients to meet their own attachment needs. (See Chapter 4 Technique #9: Healing the Inner Child.)

TECHNIQUE #7: Maintaining Boundaries

Description: Be warm but firm with boundaries. Give advanced notice about vacation and remind the patient.

Rationale: The patient may have experienced boundary violations in the past. They might not know how to keep boundaries. The therapist keeps boundaries to help the patient feel safe and demonstrate what appropriate boundaries look like.

Script: I would like to hear about that, but we are out of time for today. We are scheduled to see each other next week, and it is important, so we will be sure to address it next week.

The therapist uses a warm voice, but a firm body language (sit straight up.)

TECHNIQUE #8: Safety

Description: Help the patient feel safe with self-regulation and exploring what's stressing them.

Rationale: Address safety early on to reduce or prevent further traumatization. Patients need to feel safe before they'll open up and start exploring. It's hard to self-regulate when there's still ongoing safety issues and the patient is in fight or flight mode. Regulation creates a sense of safety. It allows the patient to be calm enough to think and feel. It lets the patient know that this is not too much for the patient and therapist to handle.

Note: Address safety within the session and outside of the session, including the patient's work, home, and other interpersonal relationships. There's safety in predictability and boundaries.

Script: What's stressing you (e.g., suicide, self-harm, physical illness, aggression, legal issues?)

What can you do to feel safe?

Let's take a moment to do a self-regulation skill.

TECHNIQUE #9: Slowing Down the Process

Description: Slow down the process to co-regulate and create containment.

Rationale: The patient needs space to talk, process, and understand what happened to them. They need to stay in the present, and tolerate their emotions and body sensations.

Note: Validate the patient's desire to get the story out, then slow down and work through what happened. Help patients use grounding and regulation skills. The patient may need redirection when they're disorganized and dysregulated.

Script: I understand that you are eager to get the story out. However, I'm having difficulty following your story. You're getting disorganized. I sense your distress.

(If the patient is numb or dissociated, in other words not in the window of tolerance, the therapist can redirect the patient's attention to their feelings by saying, "I'm feeling upset even just hearing about this. How are you feeling?")

Let's slow down. It's important that you're able to tolerate this and regulate your emotions. Let's do an exercise to get regulated.

TECHNIQUE #10: Choice

Description: Give the patient as much choice as possible.

Rationale: Give the patient power and control back and also guide them in the right action. Having a sense of agency can help patients take action. It aids them in distinguishing between the present, where they have choice, versus the past, when they didn't have choice or control.

Note: Choices can be simple, so the patient doesn't feel overwhelmed.

Script: Where would you like to sit (or where would you like me to sit?)

What do you want to talk about first?

When do you want to do your homework? Do you want to start it before lunch or dinner? (The requirement is for the patient to do their homework, but they have a choice about when.)

I think of therapy as a journey to Rome. "All roads lead to Rome," so there are many different paths that we can take. You pick the one that makes sense for you.

TECHNIQUE #11: Curious

Description: Be curious and try the exercise.

Rationale: Help patients commit to simple choices and be curious rather than judgmental. Patients who have been traumatized can be indecisive, They fear making decisions and failure.

Script: Let's try it and see what happens.

TECHNIQUE #12: Validation

Description: Provide appropriate validation.

Rationale: Validation helps patients make sense of their feelings, thoughts, and behaviours, and communicates acceptance. The first trauma is the event that happened. Further traumatization occurs after the initial trauma when people around the patient are mis-attuned, invalidating or do not allow the patient to debrief about what happened. Therefore, the second trauma is traumatic invalidation.

Note: Validation isn't praise or reassurance. Patients need time to accept the validation or accept that they were abused or traumatized. The process of accepting validation is part of the therapy. Validate what is valid, but not the bad behaviour. Validate: Emotions, thoughts, desires, difficulty / struggles, and what is effective. Be open-minded, nonjudgmental, and don't make assumptions about the patient's motives.

Caveat: Empathy, compassion, and closeness can be triggering. If the patient is getting triggered, be more matter-of-fact and less emotional. The therapist can say, "How are you doing? Are you with me? Is this too much? Let's do an exercise to regulate together." People invalidate their own experiences. They rush to put it behind them or pretend they are okay.

Script: It makes sense that you feel frustrated. You find it challenging to deal with interpersonal conflicts. At the same time, punching people is not an acceptable behaviour. (Validate the frustration that the patient feels. Don't validate punching people. There are vulnerable emotions underneath an anger outburst.)

TECHNIQUE #13: Balancing between Validation and Challenge

Description: Balance being supportive and empowering patients.

Rationale: Validation can help the patient feel heard. Once the patient is in the window of tolerance, challenge them to reflect on their behaviour and create alternative responses.

Script: E.g., Patient yelling at the receptionist.

Therapist: It is frustrating to wait so long. It is okay to feel frustrated, but not okay to yell in the office.

What would be a more helpful behaviour?

TECHNIQUE #14: Secrecy and Truth Telling

Description: Help patients find language for the secrets and what was forbidden.

Rationale: Patients sometimes doubt their own reality, because they were told lies and the experience was confusing (e.g., the patient was told "this is love" when the act was abusive.) Telling the truth can help reduce shame. Self-deception protects the relationship to the abusive caregiver, keeps loyalty, protects the image / "saves face," and preserves the status quo. Patients can fear the consequences of speaking up, e.g., becoming an outcast. They may fear or want to avoid the memory or emotion because it is hard to cope with.

Note: Telling the truth and labelling it trauma can be validating because it says that the trauma was real and it was not the patient's fault. "I'm a trauma survivor," becomes part of the patient's identity. Medical diagnosis such as Borderline Personality Disorder can be unhelpful when speaking with the patient because it can be seen as blaming the patient. Instead, labelling it as trauma and discussing recovery can be more helpful.

Script: What purpose did keeping secrets serve?

Why is it important to be able to tell the truth?

What do you think the trauma says about you? (Memory / thoughts + emotion + meaning lead to growth. Notice shame. Revealing the secret reduces shame.)

How are you feeling now that you have shared this? Has anything changed or felt different? (Notice how the feeling may change between sessions. Different parts of the patient may have different feelings about the event.)

What does sharing this with me mean to you? (See Knowledge #8: Step 2 Discussing the Relationship. Sometimes the shame will activate the patient's attachment system.)

TECHNIQUE #15: Resistance

Description: Working with resistance.

Rationale: Change can be scary, so patients resist change and therapy techniques.

Note: Sometimes the therapist needs to radically accept that the patient might not be ready to change certain things or follow a specific recommendation at this point.

Script: Why not just give up? (Be a devil's advocate.)

You worry more at a specific time of the day, but don't worry at other times. Save all the worry for those, e.g., fifteen minutes. (Prescribe the problem behaviour for a specific time.)

If you have been dissociating, not listening, and avoiding participation, double the effort. Really dissociate, really avoid listening, and really avoid the participation. (Instruct the opposite.)

Therapist: I can see that you're feeling frustrated. It takes practice to get good at using the skill. (Validate.) Can you describe to me what you did? (Review what was done.)

Patient: I touched the ice to my forehead, but it didn't work for distress tolerance. (See Chapter 1 Technique #9: Diver's Reflex.)

Therapist: How long did you do it for?

Patient: Just a few seconds.

Therapist: Try holding the ice to your face and tip of your nose for longer. Did you try any of the other techniques we went over?

Patient: No.

Therapist: What made it difficult to do the homework?

Patient: I just got busy and forgot.

Therapist: What can you do to remind yourself?

Patient: Set a reminder.

Therapist: How will you do this?

Patient: I'll put a reminder on my phone.

Therapist: How committed are you to doing this on a scale of one to ten?

Patient: Three.

Therapist: What can we do to get you to a four? What are your goals?

TECHNIQUE #16: Contradicting Behaviour

Description: Working with patients who act in contradicting ways.

Rationale: Traumatized patients sometimes compartmentalize and have difficulty mentalizing, so they act in contradicting ways.

Note: Notice ambivalence. Help identify a patient's goals and their different feelings about their goals.

Script: I am hearing that you want two very opposite things (bring mindful attention to it.) I notice that you are acting in very opposite ways.

For example, you said you want to live for as long as possible; then you said if you had a gun, you would shoot yourself.

Can you help me understand where these opposite statements are coming from? Now allow the different parts of you to discuss amongst themselves and come up with what you most want. (See Chapter 5 Technique #17: Ambivalence / Working with Parts.)

TECHNIQUE #17: Avoidance

Description: Address Avoidance.

Rationale: Patients can be ambivalent about opening up and telling their story. Some patients use avoidance to regulate their emotions. Patients are more likely to open up in a safe environment and when they are in their window of tolerance.

Note: Pay attention to losses and shame. Shame makes people hide. For patients who have difficulty feeling safe, try using Chapter 4 Technique #2: Imagining Personal Bubble. If a patient has difficulty self-monitoring triggering events, the therapist can help identify them.

Script: Therapist: I notice that when we start talking about your family, you change the topic very quickly, and sometimes you are not answering the question. I am curious about what may be going on.

Patient: I just don't like talking about it. I wish my divorce had gone differently. I should have tried harder.

Therapist: What feelings are coming up for you now?

Patient: Disappointment.

Therapist: I also sense that there is some shame and feeling of loss. Is this accurate?

Patient: Yes.

Therapist: Would you like to work on these emotions?

Patient: Sure.

Therapist: (See Chapter 7 Technique #8: Shame and Self-blame, and Chapter 4 Technique #12: Funeral of the Broken Dreams.)

TECHNIQUE #18: Exploring Fears About the Relationship

Description: Openly discuss possible fears that may come up regarding the therapeutic relationship.

Rationale: Provide psychoeducation about the fears and co-create a plan in case these fears arise.

Note: Apply ABCs of CBT to the situation.

Script: The following fears may happen during therapy. Let's discuss the possible situations and how you may feel, think, and behave. How would you like me to respond?

Situations:

- If I open up and feel emotionally close to my therapist...
- If negative emotions come up for me during the therapy, such as anger...
- If my therapist cannot meet my expectations...

Situation	Affect / Feel	Behave	Cognition / Think	Preferred Therapist Response
	I may feel...	I may behave...	I may think...	I would like my therapist to respond by...

Addressing Traumatic Re-enactment

Traumatic re-enactment occurs when the therapist gets triggered. This is the interaction between the patient and the therapist's attachment.

KNOWLEDGE #6: Step 1 Therapist Mentalizing

The therapist observes self, mentalizes, and is curious, self-compassionate, and nonjudgmental.

Therapist asks self:

- What state of mind am I in? (See Chapter 2 State of Mind.)
- What are my needs: wanting to be liked, successful, useful, or to avoid conflict?

- What triggered me or what activated my attachment system? Why now?
- What are my vulnerabilities? What am I trying to protect myself from?
- What am I feeling? Why do I hate this patient? (Notice countertransference.)
- What triggered my patient?
- What are my patient's fears? (The patient may fear that the therapist will abandon them, get angry, hurt them, give up, or loosen the boundary with the patient.)
- How did I deal with this previously?
- How did I act or react? (Notice making exceptions or breaking rules for the patient.)
- What new responses can I make?

Note: Therapist to get peer supervision and support.

KNOWLEDGE #7: Step 2 Discussing the Relationship

Discuss the therapeutic relationship during the therapy in a timely way. Be curious. Provide containment and explore.

The therapist can:

- Notice the conflict: "I am curious about what you and I are experiencing."
- Call it conflict: "You and I are having a conflict."
- Invite the discussion: "I'm hoping to discuss this together."
- Be curious: "I'm wondering what triggered you during our work together."
- Understand the patient's perspective and demonstrate active listening skills. (See Chapter 6 Technique #10: Active Listening.)

- Discuss the experience and stay in the present: "You feel... when I did..." Notice the missing emotion and help the patient reconnect to it. "What was difficult about crying in front of me? How did that make you feel?"
- Validate the patient. (See Chapter 8 Technique #12: Validation.)
- Explore the patient's prior relationships. People have the tendency to repeat old relationship patterns. This is different from the patient's previous relationships. "What were your prior experiences when you opened up to others?" "What happened when you relied on other people in the past?"
    - E.g., The therapist hears from the nurse that the patient complained to her that the therapy was very unhelpful and he wants to complain to the College. Therapist: "I am sorry that you felt the therapy was unhelpful. You sounded really upset. I'm wondering what happened that made you feel this way. I am curious about what I can do differently to support you."

KNOWLEDGE #8: Step 3 Repairing the Relationship

Relationships require work. Patients who have "personality disorders" experience challenges with relationships. That said, relationships can be repaired (see below). Help the patient develop other healthy relationships in their life. (See Chapter 6.)

TECHNIQUE #20: Addressing Misinterpretations

Description: Explore and address misinterpretations.

Rationale: Patients from dysfunctional households would try to guess the mood in the home when they were children. They tried to mentalize, and sometimes they jumped to incorrect conclusions about other people's thoughts or feelings.

Case: The patient put a plastic bag over her head as a suicidal gesture. After the nurse de-escalated the patient, the patient then said to the nurse, "I think my therapist is going to be pissed when she finds out."

Script: Therapist: I want you to take a good look at my face and tell me if I looked pissed.

Patient: No.

Therapist: How do you think I'm actually feeling right now?

Patient: No idea.

Therapist: What I am feeling is concerned and worried. I am worried that you will hurt yourself. What does this tell you about your perceptions of how other people are feeling?

Patient: I am wrong.

Therapist: Sometimes our guesses about how the other person is feeling are incorrect, and we can find out about how the other person is feeling by asking them.

Patient: (Nods.)

Therapist: I am curious about what happened that led you to putting the plastic bag over your head.

TECHNIQUE #21: Therapist as Perpetrator

Description: Address the therapist behaving like the perpetrator: being angry or harsh with the patient.

Rationale: The therapist feels hurt and loses empathy.

Note: Sometimes the therapist makes exceptions for the patient then tries to reinforce rules. (The therapist goes from being the rescuer to perpetrator.) Notice how you feel as the therapist:

angry, disappointed, or anxious. It's important for the therapist to empathize and be consistent with boundaries.

Case: The patient first asks for virtual appointments to better fit their schedule. The patient then goes from doing virtual sessions at home to meeting in their car in a noisy setting and coming to appointments late. The patient becomes progressively later for the appointments. The therapist feels disrespected and gets angry at the patient.

Script: Address therapy interrupting behaviours early. (See Chapter 8 Technique #6: Therapy-disrupting Behaviour.)

Therapist: I would like to review the contract that we signed and the expectations of therapy. (See Chapter 8 Technique #3: Sample Contract.)

Let's review your goals and priorities for therapy. (See Chapter 8 Technique #5: Priorities and Aligning Goals / Getting Buy-in.)

TECHNIQUE #22: Therapist as Victim

Description: Address the therapist becoming the victim and the patient behaving like a perpetrator.

Rationale: The therapist feels anxious when seeing the patient because they fear aggressive behaviour. The patient pushes the therapist away for self-protection, because they fear being vulnerable and therefore want to strike first.

Note: The therapist can leave if they feel unsafe. Help the patient regulate their emotions and be self-compassionate about the patient's vulnerability.

Script: E.g., The patient stands up and starts yelling and swearing during therapy.

Therapist: I feel unsafe when you start yelling and swearing. I need you to sit down and lower your voice. I will leave if I continue to feel unsafe. (Give warning.)

Patient then smashes a mug. Therapist leaves.

Next session.

Therapist: I want to explore what happened during our last session. In order for us to continue working together, this needs to be a safe space for both of us.

Patient: I was just PISSED OFF.

Therapist: I can see that and I also sense that you are feeling angry again. Let's do an exercise to regulate our emotions. (Use Stage 1 Skills.) How are you feeling now?

Patient: Less angry.

Therapist: Who are you feeling angry towards?

Patient: At the person who abused me, and at myself.

Therapist: It makes sense to be angry at the abuser. Tell me more about the anger that you feel towards yourself.

Patient: I should have done a better job of protecting myself and my sister.

Therapist: If you had a friend who had undergone the same experience as you, what would you say to the friend? (Challenge hot thoughts. See Chapter 5.)

TECHNIQUE #23: Therapist as Rescuer

Description: Address the therapist becoming the rescuer with the patient as the victim.

Rationale: The therapist wants to protect the patient and fix things quickly. The therapist tells the patient what to do instead of empowering the patient and giving them choices. The patient feels the therapist is their only hope. The therapist is working harder than the patient. The patient is using the defence response Attach and Cry for Help. (See Chapter 9 Knowledge #15f.)

Note: Empower the patient to meet their own needs rather than rely on repeated validation and reassurance from the therapist.

Script: E.g., The therapist tells the patient to leave an abusive household.

Therapist: What are the pros and cons of staying in that household? (See Chapter 2 Technique #11: Pros and Cons.)

Part of you wants to remain in the household, but another part of you wants to get out and knows that you can get seriously hurt if you stay. (See Chapter 5 Technique #17: Ambivalence / Working with Parts.)

E.g., Patient needs frequent reassurance and has difficulty making decisions.

Explore their values. Help them set boundaries, goals, and problem solve. Increase their sense of mastery and self-esteem. (See Chapter 3 Techniques #7-12.)

Empower the patient to meet their own needs. (See Chapter 4 Technique #9: Healing the Inner Child.)

TECHNIQUE #24: Therapist as Bystander

Description: Address the therapist being a bystander: not speaking up when seeing self-harming, therapy interrupting behaviour.

Rationale: Help the therapist challenge and validate the patient to promote insight and growth. (See Chapter 8 Technique #13: Balance Between Validation and Challenge.)

Note: The therapist may be a bystander because they feel resigned or lose hope and do not challenge the patient.

Script: The patient brings in their journal and reads lengthy entries to the therapist, taking up most of the session, and leaving no time for discussion or for the therapist to speak.

Therapist: I am going to stop you. I know that you are eager to share your journaling. At the same time, I noticed that for the last few sessions, your journaling has taken up most of the session, which leaves us almost no time to discuss the contents. I am wondering what is going on.

What are you getting out of this?

How can we better balance the time spent in therapy?

Summary

The therapeutic relationship is critical for recovery. It helps the patient trust and believe in the therapist and give them influence and charm. Regardless of whether the patient explicitly provides a trauma history, using a trauma-informed approach universally helps to facilitate recovery. Each insecure attachment type presents unique challenges. When a therapist finds a patient "challenging," it is important to mentalize and think about attachment types and traumatic re-enactments. Discuss the therapeutic relationship during the therapy and explore the challenges with the patient in a timely fashion. Be attuned to the patient, model healthy interactions, and co-regulate with the patient. In doing so, the therapeutic relationship can provide containment and safety. Once patients feel safe and emotionally regulated, they can then explore the world and themselves, and understand and process information. The therapeutic relationship is a powerful tool that can be used to heal attachment disorders.

CHAPTER 9:
Psychological Trauma

This chapter provides definitions of trauma and trauma-related concepts: adverse childhood events, PTSD, developmental trauma, complex PTSD, toxic stress, moral injury, and dissociation. The connection between trauma, psychological and physical symptoms, and addiction are explored. Traumatized patients can be easily triggered by trauma reminders, and they often get stuck in defence responses. Techniques to address this are provided. Psychoeducation helps the patient understand their symptoms. Breaking up trauma treatment into three steps gives the therapist an organized approach to treatment.

KNOWLEDGE #1: What is Trauma

Trauma overwhelms the brain's ability to process and integrate the experience. People get stuck in the trauma as if it was continuing to happen, because they cannot integrate the information and experience. Trauma is not "just an event" or a memory. It is a reaction to an overwhelming experience. It has ongoing impacts on people's cognition, emotions, behaviour, relationships, and physiology. Trauma affects perception; people who are traumatized perceive the world as dangerous, and this creates ongoing stress.

Different people experience the same event differently, so what is traumatic for one person is not necessarily traumatic for another, and vice versa. It depends on the person's resources, resilience, and ability to cope.

KNOWLEDGE #2: Multigenerational Trauma

Trauma can be transmitted from the people who are traumatized to their children. There are different possible reasons why trauma might be passed down. Trauma affects parenting and social behaviours. Children learn from and mirror their parents. The parent's attachment style can impact the children's attachment styles. Epigenetics can be affected and passed down.

For example, many of Canada's Indigenous people experienced traumatic events at residential schools. They were separated from their parents, culture, and language. When children who experienced this level of disconnection and loss as well as trauma became parents, they may have struggled due to not having been able to grow up in a family environment or with loving care-givers. Trauma and dislocation from family affects parenting. The effect of stress on epigenetics can also be passed to the next generation.

KNOWLEDGE #3: Adverse Childhood Experiences (ACEs)

Felitti et al. looked at ACEs and their impact on health risk behaviours and diseases.

A greater number of ACEs correlated with:

- Increased risk of mental illnesses, including: substance abuse, depression, and suicide attempts
- Increased risk of physical illness, including: sexually transmitted disease, obesity, fractures, cancer, heart disease, lung disease, and liver disease

ACEs:

- Neglect: emotional, physical
- Abuse: emotional, physical, sexual
- Dysfunctional home: parental divorce or separation, witnessing domestic violence, or having a household

member with substance abuse problems, incarceration, or mental illness

Not looked at in the original study but still impactful:
- Bullying, substandard schools or abusive teachers
- Discrimination and racism
- Community violence, assault
- Loss of a parent
- Natural disasters
- Accidents
- Poverty, homelessness
- Foster care
- Juvenile justice system

Note: ACEs do not usually result in PTSD.

KNOWLEDGE #4: Positive Childhood Experiences

Bethell C et al. and Narayan A et al. looked at how positive childhood experiences help build resilience, including:
- Positive relationships: Supportive family, another caregiver or adult, friend, teacher, or neighbour
- Positive environment: Predictable home routine, enjoyable school, enjoyable community tradition, and opportunities for good times

Note: See Chapter 3 Technique #15: Building Resilience.

KNOWLEDGE #5: Toxic Stress / Chronic Stress

Toxic stress is stress that is prolonged, or that occurs too often and quickly for the person to adapt to or recover from.

Stress leads to mobilization of defence action. However, if there is immobilization, such as not being able to escape, and the defence action cannot be carried out or is ineffective, the patient shuts down.

KNOWLEDGE #6: Moral Injury

Moral injury occurs when people witnessed, failed to prevent, or did something that is contradictory to their moral beliefs or values. This causes distress and they may feel betrayed by their peers or leaders. They may also feel angry, guilty, shameful, disgusted, worthless, unloved, or unlovable.

E.g., Veterans killing civilians in war.

E.g., Health care workers not being able to help patients.

People can suffer from both moral injury and PTSD. Having moral injury in addition to PTSD can worsen symptoms, including increased depression, suicidal thoughts, and lower functioning.

KNOWLEDGE #7: PTSD

Some people who experience trauma will go on to develop PTSD. The diagnosis of PTSD is given to patients who meet a specific set of DSM-5 diagnostic criteria.

The patient has a traumatic experience and has the following symptoms:
- Re-experiencing
- Avoidance
- Negative mood and cognition
- Hyperarousal

The symptoms last more than one month, impair function, or cause distress, and are not due to medication, substances, or another illness.

The PTSD Checklist (PCL-5) is a twenty item checklist that can be used to screen for PTSD and monitor PTSD symptoms.

Structured interviews used for diagnosing PTSD include:
- Adults: Clinician-Administered PTSD Scale for DSM-5 (CAPS-5), Structured Clinical Interview for the DSM-5 (SCID-5).
- Children: Trauma Symptom Checklist, The University of California at Los Angeles Post-traumatic Stress Disorder Reaction Index for DSM-5 (UCLA PTSD-RI-5).

Risk factors for developing PTSD after trauma: Being alone and unsupported after trauma, history of prior trauma and / or adverse childhood event, past history or family history of psychiatric illness, poor education, low socioeconomic status, physical injury during trauma, and severe emotional reaction to the trauma.

KNOWLEDGE #8: Developmental Trauma Disorder (DTD)

Dr. Bessel van der Kolk et al. proposed the diagnosis of DTD for early or childhood trauma that occurred at critical periods when the child's brain and body were developing. It can create a psychopathology that is not well captured with the current PTSD diagnostic criteria.

Attachment disorder plus trauma:
- Dysregulated mood and physiology
- Dysregulated attention and behaviour
- Dysregulated self and relationship

In other words, toxic stress plus interpersonal trauma and lack of a supportive adult leads to psychopathologies. Trauma and disorganized attachment in particular lead to major psychopathologies. Patients with disorganized attachment are more likely to dissociate. Dissociation before or around traumatic events increases the risk of developing PTSD. On the other hand, having a supportive and attuned adult helps the child regulate, tolerate, and integrate difficult experiences, allowing them to recover and grow.

KNOWLEDGE #9: Complex Trauma (CT)

Complex Trauma includes developmental trauma, but doesn't always have roots in childhood. CT can also develop in adults who experience multiple, prolonged, or severe trauma. These traumatic experiences are often invasive and interpersonal trauma, such as torture, sex trafficking, war, etc.

Symptoms of CT:
- Dysregulated mood and behaviour, which can put the patient at risk for further traumatization
- Dissociation
- Deficits in attention and concentration, difficulty with information processing and executive function, including difficulty filtering out relevant versus irrelevant information, and perceived threats in non-threatening situations
- Interpersonal difficulties, issues with boundaries and trust
- Difficulty with a sense of self and distorted expectations of the world

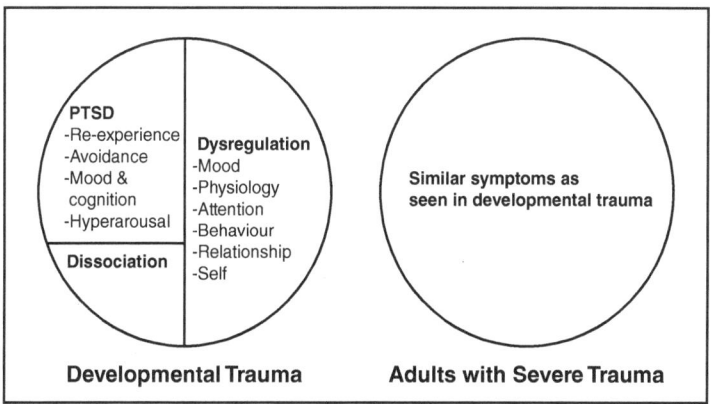

Figure 5: Complex Trauma

KNOWLEDGE #10: Pathological Self-Soothing / Addiction

When patients seek ways to cope with the emotional dysregulation, they may develop pathological self-soothing mechanisms or addictions. Addiction is a secondary problem, to deal with the primary problem of emotional pain from trauma.

Addictions provide both short-term relief from the pain and escape from the harsh reality, but are detrimental in the long run. Addiction can lead to further traumatization. Patients have difficulty giving the addiction up, or feel out of control, given the quick reward it provides.

Treatment helps people tolerate and regulate their emotions, rather than suppress and escape from them. Assist patients in finding ways to express their pain so they can heal from the trauma that's causing their suffering.

Example of pathological self-soothing:
- Substances including alcohol, tobacco, marijuana
- Abusing prescription medications or over-the-counter medication
- Food
- Self-harm
- Workaholism
- Adrenaline junkie
- Gaming, gambling
- Shopping, hoarding
- Sex, porn

What addiction does for people:
- Avoids negative emotions and feelings: Escape, relief, numbness, distraction, or disconnection
- Achieves positive emotions, feelings, and experiences: Feel high, alive, free, complete; boost self-esteem, or sleep

Other behaviours that patients may engage in to cope with trauma include avoidance, safety seeking, and overly controlling.

KNOWLEDGE #11: Dissociation

Dissociation is disconnection of:

- Consciousness
- Memories (dissociative amnesia)
- Emotions (numb)
- Identity or self (dissociative identity)
- The surrounding environment (derealization)
- Perception (of time and space)
- The body (depersonalization)

Dissociation is a coping strategy that allows patients to escape from intolerable experiences. It can be brought on by traumatic reminders or stress. Dissociation interferes with learning. People can have varying degrees of awareness about dissociation.

KNOWLEDGE #12: Trauma's Impact on Physical Body and Disease

In addition to affecting thoughts, behaviour, feelings, attention, and social connections, trauma also affects the body.

Note: Also see Knowledge #3: ACEs.

Chronic stress increases cortisol, adrenaline, and inflammatory cytokines. This affects:

- Immune system (autoimmune disease and atopy): Eczema, psoriasis, asthma, allergies, thyroid diseases
- Cardiovascular: Heart attack, stroke, elevated BMI, dyslipidemia, insulin resistance
- Gastrointestinal: IBS

- Pain perception: Chronic pain, fibromyalgia, chronic headache or migraine, arthritis, back pain, interstitial cystitis
- Chronic fatigue
- Cancer
- More medically unexplained symptoms

KNOWLEDGE #13: Somatoform Dissociation

DSM-5's dissociative disorders emphasize psychological dissociation, but somatoform dissociation is touched upon in the DSM-5's conversion disorder and somatization section.

A score of higher than thirty on the Somatoform Dissociation Questionnaire (SDQ) is significant for somatoform dissociation.

- Motor:
    - Loss of motor control: Paralysis, weakness, aphonia
    - Motor symptoms: Pseudoseizures, spasms / tics / contracture
- Sensory:
    - Loss of sensory: Loss of sensation or touch / unable to feel pain, blindness, deafness
    - Sensory symptoms: Unexplained pain, pain out of proportion, medically unexplained symptoms, somatic complaints

Conversion disorder is more frequently seen in soldiers or childhood sexual abuse survivors. Patients with pseudoseizures are more likely to have a history of child abuse (including incest abuse) than patients with epilepsy.

KNOWLEDGE #14: When to Consider DTD and CT

Although DTD and CT are not diagnoses in the DSM-5, they are useful concepts. ICD-11 has complex PTSD (cPTSD) as a diagnosis.

Without the concept of DTD / CT or diagnosis of cPTSD, patients with this clinical picture often get multiple diagnoses or get different diagnoses from different clinicians.

Given the widespread impact of trauma as discussed above and current limitations of the DSM-5, patients with trauma may be diagnosed with:

- Trauma and Stressor-Related Disorders: PTSD, Reactive Attachment Disorder, Disinhibited Social Engagement Disorder
- Mood disorders
- Dissociative disorders
- Somatoform dissociation: Conversion disorder, somatization, medically unexplained symptoms ("not yet diagnosed")
- Disorders with relational issues: Personality disorders (especially BPD, also Cluster B and or C), Autism Spectrum Disorder, Oppositional Defiant Disorder
- Attentional issue: ADHD
- Addictive behaviours: Non-suicidal self-injury, eating disorders, substance abuse
- Dysregulated physiology: Insomnia Disorder
- Disorders with behavioural issues: OCD (washing hands / body, feeling disgusted with self), Conduct Disorder, Intermittent Explosive Disorder

Think about undiagnosed trauma when:
- Things don't make sense
- The patient makes you feel confused or inadequate

- Patients are dysregulated or suicidal
- Multiple "not-yet-diagnosed" diagnoses
- Multiple psychiatric diagnoses +/- multiple medical diagnoses
- Functionally much older and sicker than others their age

KNOWLEDGE #15: Defence Responses

Defence responses activate when people are threatened, to help them act and survive. However, traumatized patients can get stuck in these defence responses when they are no longer applicable to the current situation. Sometimes the patient was unable to complete this response due to trauma, so they got stuck. These responses affect the therapeutic relationship and can play into traumatic re-enactment. (See Chapter 8 Knowledge #3: Traumatic Re-enactment.) Use Stage 1 Skills to help patients get back into the Window of Tolerance.

Note: Dr. Walter Cannon coined "fight or flight response" and other experts added additional defense responses.

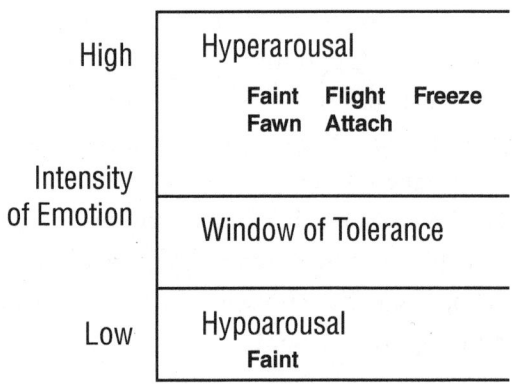

Figure 6: Defence Response and Window of Tolerance

#15a: **Fight**

Survival purpose: Defend and combat threat.

Stuck:

Action	Body Sensation	Cognition	Emotions
Aggression directed outward: Punch, kick, push, curse or yell. Blame, criticize, complain. Self-righteous. Aggression directed inward: Self-loathing, self-harm.	Heart palpitations, shortness of breath, sweaty, clenched fists / jaws, flushed.	It's their fault. It's my way or no way. I hate myself. That person did not respond to my email right away, so he must hate me (jumping to conclusions).	Anger or agitation.

#15b: **Flight**

Survival purpose: Escape and avoid threat.

Stuck:

Action	Body Sensation	Cognition	Emotions
Exit-seeking. Using addiction to escape (See Knowledge #10: Pathological Self-soothing / Addiction.)	Heart palpitations, shortness of breath, sweaty, jittery.	If I make a mistake, no one will ever want to hire me (catastrophize).	Anxious.

#15c: Freeze

Survival purpose: Immobilize.

Stuck:

Action	Body Sensation	Cognition	Emotions
Scan for danger. Not speak up. Not defend self. Avoid social engagements / relationships. Procrastinate.	Heart palpitations, muscle tightness, breath holding, eyes wide open.	Mind blank.	Anxious. Shame about inaction.

#15d: Faint (Collapse / Submit)

Survival purpose: Shut down to conserve energy. The body's last defence response.

Stuck:

Action	Body Sensation	Cognition	Emotions
Giving up. Using addiction to numb. (See Knowledge #10: Pathological Self-soothing / Addiction.) Avoiding social engagements / relationships.	Slow heart rate, cold, pain, heavy, limp Dissociate / numb, robotic / mechanical.	I'm worthless. I'm a victim. I can't do it. I can't refuse. Mind blank.	Indifferent / numb / apathetic. Depressed. Hopelessness. Shame. Suicidal.

#15e: Fawn (Please / Appease)

Survival purpose: Avoid conflict, make the enemy trust and feel optimistic in order to reduce abuse.

Stuck:

Action	Body Sensation	Cognition	Emotions
Comply. Self-sacrifice. Role reversal, take care of therapist.	Hunch over / shrink down.	I am a people pleaser. I don't want to disappoint. I need to keep the marriage together for the sake of my children (despite it being abusive).	Fear.

#15f: Attach / Cry for Help

Survival purpose: Call for backup.

Stuck:

Action	Body Sensation	Cognition	Emotions
Clingy, child-like behaviour. Makes frequent appointments and idealizes therapist.	Lean forward, puppy dog eyes.	Why didn't someone notice or help me? You need to save me.	Anxious. Desperate.

TECHNIQUE #1: Taking a Trauma History

Description: Take a trauma history.

Rationale: This information is valuable for linking symptoms to trauma and helps patients understand where their problems come from.

Note: Taking a trauma history might be triggering and this detail is not necessary for the treatment. Do assessment and treatment at the same time. Use Stage 1 techniques from prior chapters to help patients tolerate the emotions that come up. If a patient gets dysregulated, slow down. It's not necessary to go into the traumatic memory for treatment as there are many different ways to deal with it. However, people who are bothered by intrusive memories, or who spend lots of time avoiding traumatic reminders, will likely benefit from working with the traumatic memories.

Script: Who do you live with?

When you need help, who do you call?

When you need emotional support, who do you call?

As a child, who supported you when you needed physical help? Emotional support?

How were you disciplined as a child?

Who in the family treated you with affection?

Did you feel safe at home as a child? Who made you feel safe?

Did anyone recognize you as special?

How did your parents resolve disagreements?

When was your first sexual experience?

How did you feel about school as a child? How was your relationship with the other kids at school?

What were you good at? What accomplishments were you proud of as a child? (Competence protects against trauma. See Chapter 9 Knowledge #4: Positive Childhood Experiences.)

Variation A: Use the ACE Questionnaire

Note: Can also ask about traumatic experiences outside of the ACEs. (See Chapter 9 Knowledge #3: ACEs.)

Script: If it is alright with you, I would like to ask you ten yes-or-no questions based on your childhood experiences. These questions may bring up upsetting memories. If this happens, please let me know. We don't need to go through it all. This may be helpful in understanding where some of your problems and symptoms are coming from. Is it alright if we go through this?

Then go through the ACE Questionnaire.

TECHNIQUE #2: Psychoeducation

Description: Provide psychoeducation about the effects of trauma and put it in the context of the patient's symptoms. Set up the time frame and expectation of treatment.

Rationale: Psychoeducation helps the patient understand that it is normal and legitimate to have certain reactions and symptoms after trauma. It helps the patient understand their symptoms and teaches them coping skills to make this more manageable.

Note: The explanation will vary and needs to be modified depending on the patient's symptoms.

Script: A lot of times people who were traumatized by an abusive upbringing have difficulty regulating their emotions. They didn't learn the skills to self-regulate, which are taught by supportive parents. Some people learned to cope with the difficult experience by disconnecting and feeling numb. Feeling numb may also have been helpful when it wasn't safe to express emotions. You talked about alternating from feeling anxious to feeling numb. One of the things that we can work on together is helping you to acquire skills to tolerate and regulate your emotions, and to feel calm and safe. Is this something that you'd be interested in?

Sometimes people use food and substances to cope with or escape from these painful memories. However, these coping strategies can have undesirable consequences, including damaging your health. I think it is important for us to address this and to help you learn new coping strategies.

You mentioned that you're bothered by nightmares and feeling like you're reliving the past during the day. People who have experienced trauma sometimes have unintegrated memories that keep coming back intrusively in the forms of nightmares and flashbacks. Avoiding and trying to suppress these painful memories can make them worse. Avoidance can heighten the fear. It may be helpful to reprocess some of these memories so they don't bother you as much.

You also wanted to improve your relationships with your friends. We can work on interpersonal skills to help you be more successful in your relationships.

What do you think? Does this help you understand your symptoms?

TECHNIQUE #3: Psychoeducation on Triggers

Description: Provide psychoeducation regarding triggers.

Rationale: Help the patient understand what triggers are and to identify them.

Note: See Chapter 5 Anxiety Model.

Script: Triggers are things in the present that remind the person of past traumatic events. Traumatic reminders trigger survival responses, so the person reacts instinctively. Thinking is a slower process, so the patient acts without thinking.

In the past, triggers may have served the purpose of alerting people to danger and initiating quick responses, but they are no longer useful. They can lead to upsetting emotions or physical sensations that may be difficult for the patient to comprehend, especially when the current situation no longer warrants this response.

Triggers can be:

- External: Sights, sounds, smells, physical sensations, people, situations, etc.
  - E.g., The patient was punished by being locked in a small dark room as a child. Being in a small dark room now becomes a trigger.
- Internal: Thoughts, emotions, memories, bodily sensations, etc.
  - E.g., The patient was physically abused by a parent and thinking about the parent now becomes a trigger.

TECHNIQUE #4: Working with Triggers

Description: Using psychoeducation and CBT principles to address triggers.

Rationale: Psychoeducation normalizes reactions for people so they don't think they're crazy. Help patients be aware of the triggers and prepare for them. Allow patients to develop new behaviours, so they can choose how to respond to the stimulus.

Script: When you run into a traumatic trigger, it is difficult for your brain to tell the difference between actual danger versus a traumatic reminder. For people who have survived trauma, their brains have a lower threshold for sensing danger. The brain gets hijacked by the automatic response. One of the ways to address this is to observe your triggers. This helps keep the thinking brain online, so you can make decisions about how to respond.

Instead of numbing, try grounding and relaxation techniques, then choose what action you'll take.

If you know you're going to encounter a trigger, you can plan ahead, e.g., prepare yourself by doing breathing exercises. (See Chapter 1 Stage 1 Skills.)

Accept your emotions and distress. (See Chapter 7.)

Remind yourself of your skills. (See Chapter 3 Technique #15: Building Resilience.)

Apply CBT by recording antecedent (trigger), thoughts, feelings, behaviours, body sensations, and challenging hot thoughts. (See Chapter 5.)

TECHNIQUE #5: Working with the Fight Response

Description: Help the patients notice the fight response.

Rationale: By bringing mindful awareness of the fight response, the patient can then choose a different response. Carrying out the action may also help complete the fight response that was interrupted by the trauma.

Note: Fight response may lead to traumatic re-enactment. (See Chapter 8 Technique #22: Therapist Victim.) Other treatments include Chapter 7 Technique #4: Anger.

Script: Mindfully carry out the action: kick or throw a ball. Notice how your body feels and any thoughts or emotions that come up.

TECHNIQUE #6: Working with the Flight Response

Description: Help the patients notice the flight response.

Rationale: By bringing mindful awareness of the flight response, the patient can then choose a different response.

Note: Other treatments include Chapter 8 Technique #17: Avoidance.

Script: Imagine something mildly unpleasant, such as garbage on your left hand side. Now mindfully turn away from your left hand side. Notice how the action of moving away feels in your body. Notice any thoughts or emotions that come up.

For homework, try to mindfully go for a walk or run, and notice thoughts, emotions, and body sensations.

TECHNIQUE #7: Working with the Freeze Response

Description: Help the patients come out of freeze with self-compassion and mobilization.

Rationale: In freeze, the patient is outside their window of tolerance (in hyperarousal) and cannot absorb or process information.

Note: Don't respond negatively towards it. Sometimes patients have shame and self-blame about freezing. Freezing looks like: rigid muscles, tension, muteness, eyes wide, shoulders up, and body still. Distinguish between freeze versus unwillingness to speak.

Script: (Therapist to speak in a calm, soothing, and melodic voice. Eye contact and physical contact can be triggering.)

I notice you are having trouble speaking. Are you able to nod or shake your head? (Nodding and shaking your head is a procedurally learned body language, and people are usually able to do this.)

Are you really scared? Please nod or shake your head.

(If yes, do grounding, relaxation, or movement exercises.)

E.g., Let's get the body moving. Be mindful about how your body feels. (See Chapter 1 Technique #6: Mindful Movements.)

E.g., Breathing (See Chapter 1 Technique #1: Slow Outbreath.)

E.g., Let's do the Engaging the Five Senses exercises. Look around the room. Look all the way in one direction and then all the way in the other direction. Note the sense of safety in this room. (Then do Chapter 1 Technique #3: Engaging the Five Senses.)

E.g., Let's do some small movements. Let's try wiggling the fingers. (Then progress to larger movements.) Is there any action you would like to take? (See Chapter 1 Technique #18: Mindful Action with Traumatic Memory.)

(If not, consider dissociation or unwillingness to speak.)

(Once the patient is no longer frozen, discuss.) Let's discuss what happened. I think you were in the freeze response. Freezing was evolutionarily helpful to locate predators. Now it is unhelpful because people in freeze response feel information overload and are unable to process information. (Provide psychoeducation.)

Let's explore what triggered the freeze. What was going on right before?

TECHNIQUE #8: Working with the Faint Response

Description: Help patients come out of the faint response.

Rationale: Doing the opposite action can get the patient out of the faint response. (See Chapter 7 Technique #3: Opposite Action.)

Note: Persistent faint response risks further trauma because the patient is unable to engage in other survival responses (fight / flight) and is not able to notice danger cues. Sometimes it looks like treatment resistant depression.

Script: Doing the opposite action can get you out of the faint response. This includes:

- Sitting up straight
- Being assertive and present. (See Chapter 1 Mindfulness.)
- Having healthy social engagement. (See Chapter 6 IPT.)

Which of these would you like to try?

TECHNIQUE #9: Working with the Fawn Response

Description: Explore fawn and learn to say no.

Rationale: This brings mindfulness to the fawn response so the patient can practice responding differently.

Note: This response disguises hyperarousal as being social. Other treatments include being assertive and engaging in self-care. (See Chapter 3 Technique #1: Self-care.) Be careful about giving positive feedback when a patient says, "You're amazing. That was very helpful." Sometimes the patient will start giving only positive responses to the therapist to take care of the therapist.

Script: How (and when) did you learn to please people?

I am wondering if there's anything else that you would like to share with me that you have felt unable to share previously.

Let's practice saying "no."

TECHNIQUE #10: Working with the Attach Response

Description: Help patients come out of the attach response.

Rationale: Address the attach response by providing psychoeducation and discussing the relationship.

Note: This is an early defence response. This behaviour sometimes gets diagnosed as BPD rather than understood. The therapist needs to maintain boundaries to avoid traumatic re-enactment. (See Chapter 8 Technique #7: Maintaining Boundaries.) The attach response may lead to traumatic re-enactment. (See Chapter 8 Technique #23: Therapist Rescuer.)

Script:

Therapist: I noticed that you have been sending me a lot of emails recently. I am unable to meet this large demand. I am curious about what is going on with you?

Patient: I am nervous that if I get too well, I won't be able to see you anymore.

Therapist: It makes sense that you feel nervous about us eventually having to end therapy. We have previously discussed the expectations for therapy. (See Chapter 8 Technique #2: Setting Expectations.) Therapy provides you with the skills to succeed in real life; it is not a substitute for real life. Let's list the pros and cons of getting better.

Patient: (See Chapter 2 Technique #11: Pros and Cons.)

Therapist: What can you do to try and meet your needs? (Try Chapter 4 Technique #9: Healing the Inner Child.)

Stepwise Treatment

Trauma disconnects. During the trauma, patients weren't able to escape or defend themselves so the emotional information becomes useless and is painful. Patients then disconnect from the painful experience. Treatment involves reconnection and integration. It creates the conditions for people to discover themselves and open up to themselves.

Note: Dr. Judith Herman wrote about the stages of trauma recovery in her book *Trauma and Recovery* (1992).

KNOWLEDGE #16: Step 1 Stabilizing

Provide the necessary psychoeducation and establish a rapport to help patients feel safe, stay calm, and regulate their emotions. This helps patients to be able to take the initiative and responsibility for their well-being. Once patients are able to regulate their emotions and feel safe, they can begin to explore and work towards change. Help them to be present and engaged in their body.

Emotional regulation: See Stage 1 Skills (these skills also cover distress tolerance and anti-dissociation / mindfulness and body techniques.) This includes DBT, mindfulness, meditation, yoga, progressive muscle relaxation, distress tolerance, hypnosis, grounding techniques, rhythm, breath, movement, etc.

If patients have attachment disorder, that also needs to be treated. (See Chapter 8 for co-regulation, and Chapter 4 Technique #9: Healing the Inner Child or Ideal Parent Figures.)

Note: Don't rush to get the trauma history as this may be triggering for patients. Question yourself whether it is to satisfy your own curiosity. You don't need to know the details to start treatment. Expect resistance to change as change can be frightening. Name the trauma, what it is, and link it to the patient's symptoms and goals. (See Chapter 9 Technique #2: Psychoeducation.)

KNOWLEDGE #17: Step 2 Processing Memory

The problem with trauma is that it isn't just about what happened to the patient, but it also involves their reactions and ongoing issues in the present. Find out what's keeping patients stuck and address the issue that is continuing the traumatic reaction. Traumatic memories are fragmented. If the patient is ambivalent about the trauma story, a part of them wants to avoid it, but another part wants to open up. Help the patient integrate the trauma and address the avoidance, so that they can stay in the present and feel the emotions and bodily sensations. Work on telling the truth and finding language for what happened. The present is a calm, safe, supportive environment for the patient to process the past. Help the patient acknowledge that the past was real and it happened to them, but now the trauma is in the past. Allow people to think about the past compassionately, what it means, correct their cognitive distortions, and grieve.

Mentalize: Patients need to be who they are right now and reflect on what happened in the past. Help patients observe themselves and find the language to express what they feel inside. (See Chapter 2.) Be curious.

Script: What's going on? What are you feeling? What did I say that triggered you?

If patients are getting too upset, slow down. Help patients maintain day-to-day function and continue to use the coping skills from Stage 1 Skills. Patients who are experiencing too much or too little emotion (numb or dissociated) have difficulty processing, so they need to be able to tolerate the experience first.

Script: Stay with the experience and stay with me. On a scale of one to ten, how present are you now? E.g., if eight, how do we get you to a ten? What do we need to do to help you feel safe and be able to tolerate the experience?

If the patient is still too upset:

Script: You seem really upset. I'm mindful of how upsetting this is. Let's use a distress tolerance skill now. We will find time to come back to this.

Note: It is important that the patient is not reliving the past as this can be re-traumatizing. They need to be able to distinguish the past from the present. Healing is not a linear process. Patients go back and forth between steps. Usually, people take a small bite of the traumatic content, process it, regulate with Stage 1 Skills, then return to process more content.

Find out what is keeping them stuck. The patients need to know that the trauma is over and that all bad things come to an end. People who cannot integrate the traumatic memory have difficulty integrating other experiences. Feelings, personal development, and behaviour get stuck and the patient re-experiences the trauma.

See Stage 2 Skills. Other things that can help include EMDR, hypnosis, CPT, psychodynamic therapy, etc.

KNOWLEDGE #18: Step 3 Post-traumatic Growth / New Normal

Help patients reconnect and create new meaning.

Self

- Connecting with aspects or parts of self. Develop healthy self-esteem, identity, and agency / competence. (See Chapter 3.)
- Trauma makes patients feel helpless. People need to take action and apply competency and agency to combat and overcome a sense of helplessness.
- Help patients get to know all parts of themselves, develop self-compassion, be kind to themselves, and come to peace.

Emotions

- Reconnect with their emotions, being able to experience the full range and self-regulate (without using pathological self-soothing mechanisms).
- Mentalizing: Be able to think and feel at the same time. Trauma makes the cognitive, thinking brain go offline.
- Help patients learn the vocabulary to communicate what they're feeling to others.
- Address emotions that may be related to the trauma: shame, guilt, grief, anger, etc.

Body

- Feel connected to their body.
- Address somatic symptoms, chronic pain.
- Help patients move their body in ways that allow them to connect with themselves and calm themselves down.

Relationship
- Connect with others and form healthy relationships. Set boundaries, be effective in getting what they want from others, and find a sense of belonging. (See Chapter 6.)
- Help patients develop healthy, secure attachments.
- Restore healthy sexuality, and re-engage in care-taking and socializing.

Pleasure
- Find a new sense of pleasure and engagement.
- Sometimes trauma makes patients feel alive and they get addicted to the trauma. They don't feel alive doing other normal or healthy activities. Help the patient learn to be present and to enjoy feeling fully alive in the here and now. (See Chapter 3.)

Meaning and Purpose
- Find meaning, sense of purpose, and motivation. Explore morals and values. (See Chapter 3.)
- Traumatized patients lose sense of purpose, motivation, and involvement. The reward system changes and needs to be restored.

Beliefs
- Acquire positive beliefs.
- Correct for trauma-related cognition, self-limiting beliefs, and extreme beliefs. (See Chapters 5 and 7.)
- Traumatized patients have negative beliefs about themselves, relations, other people, and the world. Help balance this with positive beliefs.

Healthy Behaviours
- Address addictive behaviour.

- Be able to care for oneself.
- Regulate sleep and appetite.
- Resolve PTSD symptoms.

Patients can be discharged from care if they are functioning well, the symptoms or suffering are reduced or resolved, or their treatment goals are met.

Summary

Psychological trauma, especially complex trauma, can cause a wide range of symptoms. It is important that therapists and health professionals consider the impacts of trauma, and help patients get treatment and recover.

Therapists do not need to obtain details of trauma for treatment. It is important to meet the patient where they are at. Recovery is not linear. If the patient is overwhelmed by their experience, slow down and go back to stabilize and help the patient stay in their window of tolerance. When treating patients, play to their strengths and consider what makes them resilient, including positive childhood experiences. Trauma survivors are resilient and have the ability to recover from even the most horrific events.

CHAPTER 10:
Clinical Cases

This chapter discusses how the various techniques can be applied to different clinical cases involving patients from six years old to seniors with mild dementia. For patients outside of this range, additional strategies beyond traditional ones involving one-on-one talk therapy are also discussed.

Lastly, therapist wellness and peak performance are also addressed.

Clinical Cases

Issues	Age (in years)				
	6-11	12-17	18-25	26-64	65+
Mood	Case #5: Child with Anxiety	Case #4: Teenager with Depression	Case #12: Borderline Personality Disorder (BPD)	Case #3: Postpartum Depression	Case #1: Labile Mood in Late Life Case #2: Grief and End of Life
Physiology	Case #7: Functional Abdominal Pain			Case #16: PTSD in a Veteran	Case #6: Senior with Insomnia
Attention			Case #17: Dissociative Identity Disorder (DID)		

	Age (in years)				
Issues	6-11	12-17	18-25	26-64	65+
Behaviour		Case #8: Teenager with Eating Disorder Case #9: Teenager with Obsessive Compulsive Disorder (OCD)	Case #11: Substance Abuse Case #12: BPD	Case #16: Complex PTSD in a Veteran	Case #10: Hoarding
Relationship			Case #12: BPD	Case #3: Postpartum Depression	
Self Pathology			Case #12: BPD		
PTSD / Simple Trauma	Case #14: Dog Attack			Case #13: Acute Stress in a Refugee	
Dissociation			Case #17: DID	Case #15: Dissociation and Peripartum Mental Health	
Complex Trauma			Case #17: DID	Case #16: Complex PTSD in a Veteran	

Note: It is important to have a proper medical work-up before proceeding with psychotherapy. Medical management is beyond the scope of this book.

Dysregulated Mood

CASE #1: Labile Mood in Late Life

Case #1.1: A ninety-three-year-old male from a retirement home's assisted living section presents to the clinic with his daughter. She is concerned that he is depressed, because his mood has been labile and his motivation has been poor. He spends most of his time watching TV and receives assistance for bathing, dressing, and toileting. He does not have any prior mental health history, and there have been no recent changes in his life, including no losses.

Question A: What is an important differential diagnosis to consider and how could you differentiate this?

Discussion: New onset of "depression" in late life, especially without prior mental health history, is concerning as a symptom of dementia. New onset of "anxiety" in late life is concerning for new medical problems. Prior to treating a mental illness, make sure the patient has had an appropriate work-up for medical conditions that may mimic a mental illness. Start by taking a social history. (See Chapter 8 Technique #1: Identifying Patient Baseline.)

Screening tools: For depression: Patient Health Questionnaire (PHQ-9) and Geriatric Depression Scale (GDS). For dementia: cognitive assessments, such as Montreal Cognitive Assessment (MoCA) or Mini Mental State Examination (MMSE). For depression in patients with dementia: Cornell Scale.

A helpful question to ask: Does the patient brighten up when they see their grandchildren? A patient with depression usually remains sad, while someone with dementia usually is happier when they see their grandchildren.

Patients with depression are usually very difficult to motivate, while someone with dementia may respond well to more directive instructions. Instead of asking the patient, "Do you want to come and exercise?" say, "Come, we are going to exercise," and take the patient.

Case #1.2: The patient thought he was seventy-eight years old and could not recall what he did for a living. His daughter reports that he has university level education. He answers that his mood is "fine." The patient's GDS score was in the normal range. He was unable to complete the MoCA and got very frustrated by it. His daughter relates that this is the anger she has to deal with. She corrects him when he gets things wrong or misremembers things. For example, he thought he was managing his own finances, but his daughter reminded him that she was. He then insisted that she stop being involved with his finances. This conflict led to her feeling stressed out.

Question B: What could you do next to help support the patient and his daughter?

Note: The approach to cognitive impairment including a medical work-up is not covered in this book.

Discussion: The patient has moderate dementia, so he is too cognitively impaired for the techniques covered in this book. His mood is reactive and the conflict between them is contributing to his anger. The patient's Cornell Scale score was in the normal range. Book a separate appointment to see the daughter individually for supportive counselling.

Case #1.3: The daughter is struggling with caregiver burnout and interpersonal conflict with her father.

Question C: How can you help?

Discussion:

Strategies to Reduce Interpersonal Conflict

Therapist: Your father has a new diagnosis of moderate dementia. His memory is very poor and he is living in the past. He thought he was seventy-eight. Have you tried not challenging him when he says things that are not correct?

Daughter: Honestly sometimes I am so tired of arguing with him that I just don't bother to correct him.

Therapist: What happens when you try that?

Daughter: Nothing.

Therapist: Can you describe an example? (Be curious. See Chapter 8 Technique #11: Curious.)

Daughter: When my father said he was managing his finances and talking about what stocks he bought, I just nodded. He did not get upset.

Therapist: It seems that part of you is upset about doing that. (See Chapter 5 Technique #17: Ambivalence / Working with Parts.)

Daughter: Yes. I just feel like I'm deceiving him, and I feel bad about it.

Therapist: Your father is living in the past and in his earlier version of reality. Is correcting him helpful, and does he remember it later?

Daughter: Not at all. It just makes him angry and he does not remember it. We go through the same conversation again and again.

Therapist: Rather than believing that you're deceiving him, it may be helpful to think that he has dementia and his own mind is deceiving him. Whether or not you correct him does not change his belief. Correcting him only makes him angry. (See Chapter 3 Technique #4: Reframing.)

Caregiver self-care

Therapist: It sounds like you are burning out. It is important that you take care of yourself, so you can continue caring for your father.

Daughter: I don't have time.

Therapist: It doesn't need to take up a lot of time. Do you think you can spend five minutes a day on yourself? (See Chapter 3 Technique #1: Self-care.)

Case #1.4: The daughter stops trying to correct her father and accepts that given the father's dementia, he sometimes gets the facts wrong. (See Chapter Technique #1: Radical Acceptance.) This significantly reduces the conflicts between them. After visiting her father, she goes for a walk in a nearby park as part of her self-care. (Taking time to emotionally regulate after interpersonal interaction is also part of Chapter 6 Technique #14: Planning Ahead.) She is enjoying the time with her father a lot more.

CASE #2: Grief and End of Life

Case #2.1: An eighty-two-year-old female with mild cognitive impairment recently moved to long-term care (LTC). She was previously living independently until she had a massive heart attack, complicated by congestive heart failure and renal failure. She presents to the clinic saying that she is "fed up with life."

Question A: How would you approach this?

Discussion:

Therapist: Are you thinking of ending your life? (Address safety. See Chapter 8 Technique #8: Safety.)

Patient: I have thought about it, but it is not what a good Christian would do.

Therapist: Sometimes people do not want to artificially shorten their life and instead they want to focus on their quality of life. What are your thoughts about this?

Patient: Yes, I would like to focus on my quality of life.

Therapist: What does quality of life mean to you?

Patient: I don't know. I feel like I have no quality of life right now.

Therapist: What is important in your life right now? (See Chapter 3 Technique #7: Values.) Religion?

Patient: Yes.

Therapist: Would you like to be connected to the chaplain? (Patients who identify with religious groups may want support from their religious figure).

Patient: Sure.

Therapist: What else is important to you?

Patient: My family.

Therapist: Who are the important family members in your life? (See Chapter 6 Technique #1: Exploring Patients' Social Networks. Her feelings for these people may be what is preventing the patient from wanting to end her life.)

Note: The approach to palliative care symptom management and goals of care discussion are not covered in this book, but would be important for the family physician to address.

Case #2.2: She is bothered by intense mixed emotions of frustration, sadness, and anxiety. She understands that her medical prognosis is poor.

Question B: How would you address this?

Discussion:

Therapist: Can you tell me more about these feelings?

Patient: I am frustrated that I am stuck in long-term care.

Therapist: You lost your independence. It makes sense to feel frustrated and sad. (See Chapter 8 Technique #12: Validation.) It's a grieving process. (See Chapter 6 Technique #28: Grief.)

Patient: Yes. I also feel very nervous. I was told that I don't have very long to live, given my heart failure and kidney failure. I would not want to be on dialysis. I don't know how long I have, and this makes me anxious.

Therapist: The unknown is anxiety-provoking. At the same time, none of us lives forever. No one can predict the future. I think it is more helpful to think about how to make the most of the time we have. What do you think? (Validate the patient's feeling of anxiety, then challenge the patient to think about what could be done. See Chapter 8 Technique #13: Balancing between Validation and Challenge, and Chapter 6 Technique #20: Reframing Unhelpful Thoughts. This also shifts the patient from feeling to thinking. See Chapter 2 Technique #6: Identifying States of Mind, Balanced Perspective.)

Note: The patient could also try radically accepting that she had a heart attack and is living in LTC, or that human beings are mortal. (See Chapter 7 Technique #1: Radical Acceptance.)

Question C: When using psychotherapy with a senior with cognitive impairment, what additional modifications to the techniques may be helpful?

Discussion: (Think of the Six S's.)

- Simplify: Simplify what you say and the content you cover.
- Slower: Go at a slower pace, e.g., only teach one coping skill at a time.
- Same: Repeat the exercise.
- Social supports: Involve the family to help with the homework.
- Summary: Write down a summary of the take-home points and the homework.
- Sight and sound: Make sure the patient can see and hear. Use hearing aids, glasses, and write using large fonts.

Case #2.3: The patient gets a weekly visit with a chaplain from her denomination. She believes that "when her time comes, she will join her parents in heaven." She focuses on the important connections in her life. She enjoys the visits with her family, especially with the grandchildren. She attends regular singing groups at the LTC with another co-patient who has become a friend. (See Chapter 3 Technique #3: Positive Activities.) She feels grateful about the people she has in her life and what she has accomplished. (See Chapter 3 Technique #5: Happiness and Positives.) She enjoys the present moment rather than worrying about the future. (See Chapter 1 Technique #2: Orienting to the Present). She now feels happy, calm, and content.

CASE #3: Postpartum Depression

Case #3.1: A twenty-seven-year-old at six weeks postpartum presents feeling depressed for over a month. She has ongoing interpersonal conflict with her partner and minimal family support.

Question A: What are some screening tools for postpartum depression?

Discussion: The Ten-item Edinburgh Postnatal Depression Scale or PHQ-9.

Question B: How would you explore safety?

Discussion:

Therapist: Have you had any thoughts of ending your life, hurting yourself or the infant?

Patient: No.

Therapist: Have you had any hallucinations, such as hearing or seeing things that other people can't see?

Patient: No.

Therapist: How do you and your partner deal with conflicts?

Patient: We often start yelling at each other. Sometimes we end up just avoiding the topic altogether.

Therapist: Does the conflict ever escalate to physical violence?

Patient: No.

Therapist: How easy is it for you to resolve conflicts?

Patient: Difficult.

Note: If the therapist is worried about a child's safety, they need to involve the Children's Aid Society (CAS).

Therapist: We need to keep your child safe. As you know, this is one of the limits to confidentiality that was part of our contract. (See Chapter 8 Technique #3: Sample Contract.) Would you like to call CAS together, or would you like me to call CAS? (See Chapter 8 Technique #10: Choice.)

Question C: What are some red flags for abusive relationships?

Discussion: The partner:

- Demeans, threatens, forces, guilt-trips you, and treats you poorly, especially in private.
- Tries to isolate you, dislikes your family and friends, does not like you leaving the house.
- Is frequently angry, aggressive.
- Is very possessive and jealous.
- Is very controlling, it's his way or no way, does not take no for an answer, invades your privacy (e.g., goes through your phone).
- Only his beliefs and needs matter.
- Blames others and takes no responsibility, plays victim, does not accept criticism.
- Avoids conversations, quickly changes subjects or gives vague responses.
- Lies, cheats, denies truths.

- Contradicting and unpredictable: says one thing and does the opposite, can be very charming and nice, then the total opposite.
- Is offensive or cruel to others, creates conflicts.
- Tests people, orders people to do things at the last minute.
- Expects others to be perfect.

Case #3.2: She has mild depression and only wants therapy.

Question D: What strategies may be helpful to address the interpersonal conflict?

Discussion: Chapter 6 Technique #7: Turn-Taking / Speaker Object, and Technique #13: Self-Check-in Before and During Communication may be helpful to start with.

Note: Parent support groups may be helpful (e.g., playgroups).

Case #3.3: While treating the patient with IPT and exploring the patient's social networks and closeness circle. (See Chapter 6 Technique #1: Exploring Patients' Social Networks, and #2: Closeness Circle), you discovered that the patient grew up in a dysfunctional family. When she described the relationship with her parents, you realized that she has an insecure attachment. (See Chapter 8 Knowledge #1: Attachments / AAI.)

Question E: Why is it important to treat attachment disorder in this patient?

Discussion: The infant is more likely to develop insecure attachment when the parent has insecure attachment.

Note: When young children (less than school age) present with mental health concerns, it is important to explore attachment. The child's parents may need therapy for their own mental health, or need parenting skills.

Question F: What strategies can be used to treat the patient's attachment disorder?

Discussion:

Use Healing the Inner Child

Therapist: Some people have not experienced healthy parent-child interactions. Doing this exercise can help you create a new template for healthy interactions. Having a template for healthy interaction will also help you form a healthy secure attachment with your infant. (Then proceed with Chapter 4 Technique #9: Healing the Inner Child. Once the patient is able to do Healing the Inner Child, try the variation Imagining Ideal Parents.)

Use the Therapeutic Relationship

The therapist can use the therapeutic attachment between patient and therapist and model healthy interpersonal interactions.

Question G: How can the Imagining Ideal Parents technique potentially improve interpersonal relationships?

Discussion: The patient can use the qualities from the Imagining Ideal Parents technique to create an imaginary ideal partner. (See Chapter 4 Technique #10: Imagining Ideal Partner.) Once she knows what she wants in an ideal partner, she can use the interpersonal skills from Chapter 6 to negotiate for what she needs.

Note: The patient may benefit from couples or marital therapy.

Case #3.4: Through the therapeutic attachment with the therapist and Imagining Ideal Parents technique, the patient acquires earned secure attachment. She grieved not having a good childhood (see Chapter 6 Technique #29: Grief) and accepts she cannot change her childhood. (See Chapter Technique #1: Radical Acceptance.) She joined a parenting group and feels much more supported. She and her husband are doing couples therapy as well. They are communicating more effectively. She is getting an understanding about how they trigger each other. By doing Stage 1 Skills, she is better able to regulate her emotions, which further helps communication. She tries to understand things from her husband's perspective first and not jump to conclusions. She focuses on the problem and tries to solve it with her husband. (See Chapter 6 Technique #22: Focusing on the Problem not the Person.)

She is hopeful that she can give her child the childhood that she would have wanted. (See Chapter 3 Technique #13: Fostering Hope and Optimism.)

CASE #4: Teenager with Depression

Case #4.1: A seventeen-year-old male presents with depression and very poor motivation. His mother is concerned that his academic performance has significantly suffered since switching to e-learning due to the COVID-19 pandemic. He has been binge watching TV, then sleeping in, and not doing school work.

Question A: What strategies may be helpful?

Discussion:

Set Priorities and Align Goals (See Chapter 8 Technique #5: Priorities and Align Goal / Getting Buy-in.)

Therapist: What can I do for you?

Patient: I don't know. My mom wanted me to come.

Therapist: What do you think made your mom send you here?

Patient: She's worried about my mood and my school performance.

Therapist: How do you feel about that?

Patient: (Shrugs.)

Therapist: Are those things you want to work on?

Patient: I don't know.

Therapist: I am sensing some ambivalence. Part of you wants to address it and part of you doesn't. Is that right? (See Chapter 5 Technique #17: Ambivalence / Working with Parts.)

Patient: Yes.

Therapist: How has feeling depressed been helpful?

Patient: My mom just keeps nagging me. Being depressed helps me stay in my room and avoid her.

Therapist: So part of you wants to stay depressed to avoid the nagging. There is also a part of you that wants to stop feeling depressed.

Patient: (Nods.)

Therapist: Would all parts of you be on board if we work towards getting less nagging from your mom and helping you feel better? (Get the patient to buy-in.)

Patient: Sure.

Therapist: What does better look like for you?

Patient: I want to be less of a disappointment.

Therapist: What does being accomplished look like? (See Chapter 3 Technique #4: Reframing.)

Patient: Being able to get my homework done and get good grades.

Therapist: What is making it hard for you to do this?

Patient: I just couldn't find the motivation.

Therapist: Are there some days you have more motivation than others? (See Chapter 3 Technique #5: Happiness and Positives.)

Patient: I don't know.

Therapist: You made it to our appointment today. What did you do to find the motivation to do that?

Behaviour Activation

Therapist: Other than watching TV, what do you enjoy? (See Chapter 3 Technique #3: Positive Activities.)

Patient: I used to like riding my bike, but I haven't done that in a while.

Therapist: Do you think you can dedicate five minutes a day towards getting better?

Patient: Sure.

Therapist: Would you go out and bike five minutes a day? (See Chapter 5 Technique #15: Behaviour Activation.)

Patient: I'll try.

Therapist: On a scale of one to ten, ten being totally committed, how committed are you to doing this?

Patient: Five.

Therapist: What can we do to get you to a seven?

Improve Self-esteem (See Chapter 3 Technique #12: Self-Esteem.)

Improve Sleep (See Case #6.)

Patient: I have a hard time getting up in the morning.

Therapist: What have you tried?

Patient: I tried setting an alarm and it didn't work.

Therapist: Here are some strategies that may help. Try to schedule a fun activity in the morning right after waking so you have motivation to get up or get some light right after waking up. What would you like to try?

Patient: I can try one of those.

Therapist: Do you take naps?

Patient: Yes. I nap multiple times throughout the day.

Therapist: Sometimes people use the bed to escape emotional suffering instead of sleeping. Do you relate to this?

Patient: Yes.

Therapist: Instead of going to bed, do another activity. What could you try that may be helpful?

Patient: I can listen to music.

Note: Sometimes it is helpful to work with the parent. To use encouragement rather than criticism to motivate the child.

Case #4.2: He is limiting his naps and listening to music or going for a bike ride instead. His self-esteem has improved. He started working a part time job and wants to save enough money to eventually move out and live with his friends. (See Chapter 3 Technique #9: Setting Goals.)

CASE #5: Child with Anxiety

Case #5.1: A seven-year-old female presenting with generalized anxiety.

Question A: What strategies may be helpful for relaxation.

Discussion:

Therapist: Do you know what it means to be anxious?

Patient: Yes.

Therapist: What does your body feel when you are anxious?

Patient: I feel my chest is tight and I get butterflies in my stomach.

Therapist: Today, we will talk about what to do when you feel anxious–when you feel your chest is tight and there are butterflies in your stomach. We will do exercises together to help your body relax.

Slow Outbreath

Therapist: Let's do a breathing exercise together. The important thing is to make sure the outbreath is slow.

(See Chapter 1 Technique #1: Variation A: Progressively Longer Breaths.)

Note: Some children may want to lie down on the floor with a small toy on their abdomen. The toy will rise up and down with each breath. Other children may be uncomfortable lying down. Put their hand on the abdomen and watch it rise and fall. Get the child to demonstrate. Use praise.

Progressive Muscle Relaxation (See Chapter 1 Technique #7.)

Note: Create a comfortable environment in your office. This can be done standing up (in front of a chair or a beanbag chair), lying down, or reclining in a chair.

Imagining a Safe Place (See Chapter 4 Technique #1.)

Therapist: Let's create an imaginary safe place for you to go. Which places make you feel safe?

Note: Immigrants may want to imagine places from their home country to feel safe.

Positive Activities

Do activities that calm you. (See Chapter 3 Technique #3: Positive Activities.)

Note: Be culturally sensitive. You may suggest wellness modalities that are part of the patient's cultural background. For example, people of Chinese background may feel an interest in committing to Tai-Chi as part of their mindfulness or positive activities. (See Chapter 6 Society and Culture.)

Make Something Fun

Therapist: How can you make a small thing fun?

Case #5.2: The patient is able to relax and no longer worries about having anxiety. She understands that emotions come and go.

Dysregulated Physiology

CASE #6: Senior with Insomnia

Case #6.1: A seventy-five-year-old female presenting with insomnia. She tried a few sleeping medications, but they increased the number of falls she was having. She watches TV until 8:50 p.m. and then drinks a glass of wine and goes to bed at 9 p.m. She usually spends two hours lying in bed awake. She wakes up twice in the middle of the night for one hour each, sometimes to use the washroom. She wakes up at 7 a.m. and naps from 4 to 6 p.m.

Question A: What are strategies for sleep hygiene?

Note: Dr. Peter Hauri wrote the first book on sleep hygiene.

Discussion:

Routine
- Have the same wake up time.
- Use the washroom twice to fully empty the bladder before bed.

Relaxation
- Do a relaxation exercise starting one hour before bed (e.g., Chapter 1 Technique #7: Progressive Muscle Relaxation, and Technique #8: Tapping.)
- Shower or bathe before bed, apply lotion.
- Massage yourself.

- Exercise regularly during the day or early afternoon, but not later.
- Comfortable sleep environment, appropriate temperature, good mattress.

Stimulus Control

- Go to bed only when sleepy. (If unable to sleep, get out of bed and read a calming non-work-related book under dim light, listen to a podcast or audiobook. Sleepiness is not the same as fatigue. Sleepiness is difficulty staying awake.)
- Use the bed only for sleep and sex.
- Get out of bed within ten to fifteen minutes of wake up time.
- Consider using white noise.

Minimize or Avoid

- Caffeine, nicotine, alcohol, or other stimulants (avoid caffeine six hours before bed.)
- Naps (nap before 3 p.m. and keep it to one hour or less.)
- Reclining during the day.
- Minimize or avoid around bedtime:
    - Fluids (exception, a half glass of warm milk may help with sleep)
    - Screens (e.g., TV), exercise
    - Heavy meals (except a light snack if they tend to get hungry at night, e.g., cheese and crackers)
    - Light, noise

Note: Optimize medical causes for sleep disturbance (e.g., obstructive sleep apnea).

Question B: What is the patient's sleep efficiency?

Discussion: Get patient to record this daily:

Time spent in bed	9 p.m. to 7 a.m. = 10 hours
	4 to 6 p.m. = 2 hours
	10+2 =12 hours
Time spent awake in bed	Time to fall asleep: 2 hours
	Waking up at night: 2 x 1 hour = 2 hours
	2+2= 4 hours
Total sleep time = Time spent in bed minus Time spent awake in bed	12 - 4 hours = 8 hours
Sleep efficiency (SE) = Total sleep time divided by Time spent in bed multiply by 100%	8 / 12 = 0.67
	0.67 X 100% = 67%

Question C: How do you use sleep restriction?

Discussion: Sleep restriction improves sleep efficiency by limiting the amount of time spent in bed and helps patients feel sleepy at bedtime. Patients may feel sleepy during the day for three to four weeks.

If SE < 80%: decrease the time spent in bed by fifteen to thirty minutes.

If SE > 85%: Increase the time spent in bed by fifteen to thirty minutes.

Between 80-85%: keep the current schedule.

Pick a total sleep time of at least five hours, a bedtime before 2 a.m., and a wake up time after 5:30 a.m. Modify the schedule with the patient at each session (e.g., weekly).

E.g., Patient picks to go to bed at 10 p.m. and wake up at 7 a.m. She moves her nap to 2 p.m. and limits it to one hour.

Patient's Recording

Day #: 7

Bedtime: 10 p.m.

Time it takes to fall asleep: 1hr

Number and length of each night time waking: 1 x 1hr

Wake up time: 7 a.m.

Nap time: 2-3 p.m.

New SE

Time spent in bed	10 p.m. to 7 a.m. = 9 hours 2-3 p.m. = 1 hour Total 10 hours
Time spent awake in bed	Time to fall asleep: 1 hour Waking up at night: 1 hour Total 2 hours
Total sleep time = Time spent in bed minus Time spent awake in bed	10 - 2 hours = 8 hours
Sleep efficiency (SE) = Total sleep time divided by Time spent in bed multiply by 100%	8 / 10 = 0.8 0.8 X 100% = 80%

Note: Avoid sleep restriction in bipolar disorder as it may trigger mania. Consider reducing sleep time by fifteen to thirty minutes at a time instead. If the patient is falling asleep earlier than desired, try light exposure in the evening to delay sleep onset.

Question D: How do you apply CBT to insomnia (CBT-I)?

Discussion:

Affect	Behaviour	Cognition
Anxious, frustrated.	Watch the clock.	Either I fall asleep now or I'm going to be up all night (all or nothing thinking).
		I should be able to sleep eight hours (shoulds).
		Tonight is going to be another bad night (fortune telling).
		I can never sleep well (mental filter).
		I am an insomniac (labelling).
		If I don't sleep well, tomorrow will be a disaster (catastrophizing).
		Everything will be better if I get a good night's sleep (magical thinking).

Facts Supporting	Facts Against	Balanced Perspective
I had difficulty falling asleep yesterday.	Eight hours of sleep is an average and some people need more, some less. It is unrealistic to expect everyone to always get eight hours of sleep. I was still able to function and make it to my appointment despite not sleeping well.	I sometimes have difficulty falling asleep and the amount of sleep I get varies. I can still function even if I did not sleep well.

- Create a to-do list and write down pre-sleep thoughts to reduce cognitive workload.
- Prescribe the problematic behaviour. (See Chapter 8 Technique #15: Resistance). Create a worry list.

- Write down ways to address the worry list. (See Chapter 3 Technique #10: Problem Solving.) Keeping this sheet at the bedside can remind them that they've already done the worrying.
- Observe your thoughts and emotions without judgment. (See Chapter 2 Technique #13: Observing Emotions.)
- Do a list of pros and cons for getting out of bed if unable to sleep. (See Chapter 2 Technique #11: Pros and Cons.)

Pros	Cons
Try a new method that may work.	May get less sleep.

Radical acceptance of insomnia. (See Chapter 7 Technique #1: Radical Acceptance.)

Case #6.2: The patient is no longer taking sleeping medications or wine at bedtime. Her sleep efficiency has improved. She feels calmer and happier when bedtime comes.

CASE #7: Functional Abdominal Pain

Case #7.1: A ten-year-old male presenting with functional abdominal pain. He has had a thorough medical workup, including with specialists, and no physical abnormalities were found. He is very bothered by the abdominal pain and sometimes misses school and stays home or sees the doctor.

Question A: What needs to be explored about his environment?

Discussion: What is going on at school? Are there challenges with the teacher or bullying? Is there something that is triggering anxiety there?

Case #7.2: There are no issues with the teachers or bullying at school. He appears anxious and has difficulty talking about his emotions. He gets worried about the abdominal pain and believes that he needs to rest or see the doctor when it happens.

Question B: What are some important goals for therapy?

Discussion:

- Improve coping with anxiety and the abdominal pain.
- Improve school attendance.
- Reduce unnecessary medical appointments.

Note: The brain perceives the pain. Stress worsens pain. The patient subconsciously focuses on physical rather than emotional pain.

Question C: What strategies may be helpful?

Discussion:

Teach the Mind-Body Connection (See Chapter 1 Mind-Body Connection.)

Therapist: You have been having stomach aches and have missed school and seen many doctors because of this. The doctors have said that you are physically fine. The stomach aches are not dangerous. Different emotions have different physical feelings in our body. Let's talk about different emotions. (See Chapter 2 Technique #1: Teaching Language for Emotions.)

Anxiety can feel like stomach aches or butterflies in the stomach. Worrying about the stomach aches can worsen the anxiety and create a negative cycle. Behaviours like missing school and going to the doctor can worsen the belief that the stomach aches are something serious and make the anxiety worse. We will work on stopping this negative cycle together. Let's do some relaxation exercises (See Case #5.)

Practice Body Scan (See Chapter 2 Technique #14: Variation A: Use Body Scan for Interoception.)

CBT (See Chapter 5.)

Situation	Thoughts	Emotions and Intensity (0-100)	Body Sensation
The teacher wrote out today's homework on the board. I have a stomach ache.	There's too much to do. I can't do it all. I'll fail. My dad will be upset. The stomach ache is dangerous. I need to see a doctor right away. I need to go home and rest.	Anxious: 90.	Stomach ache. Chest tightness. Heart beating fast. Muscles tight. Dizzy.

Facts Supporting	Facts Against
Sometimes I can't finish my homework. My stomach ache makes it hard for me to get homework done.	Sometimes I finish my homework even when there's a lot. I have passed even when I didn't get all the homework done. I have been having the same stomach aches for a while and the doctors have told me they are not dangerous.

Balanced Perspective	Re-rate Affect and Intensity	Body Sensation After CBT
There's a lot of homework, but I'll try my best to get it done. My stomach aches don't feel good but are not dangerous.	Anxious: 40.	Stomach ache is better. Breathing is better.

Note: It may be helpful to add body sensation after the CBT to see if there's any improvement. It will help to reinforce the mind-body connection. When working with children, involve a supportive parent or guardian to help with the homework.

Working with Flight: Try to imagine moving towards and away from mild anxiety-provoking stimuli. (See Chapter 9 Technique #6.)

Case #7.3: The patient no longer misses school for the functional abdominal pain. He understands when he is feeling anxious and the body sensations that go with it. He can apply relaxation techniques to help improve the abdominal pain, so that it is tolerable.

Dysregulated Behaviour

CASE #8: Teenager with Eating Disorder

Case #8.1: A fourteen-year-old female presenting with an eating disorder–binge and restrict. This has become worse since she started high school this year.

Question A: What needs to be considered before starting psychotherapy?

Discussion: Medical stability. Patients, especially those with very low weight, can have medical complications and those usually need to be treated before psychotherapy.

Case #8.2: Her body weight is in the low normal range and she is medically stable.

Question B: What is body image?

Discussion: Body image is what people perceive, feel, and think about their appearance.

Question C: What strategies can help the patient develop a healthy body image and be comfortable with their appearance?

Discussion:

- Explore body image from the patient's, people in their closeness circle's, (see Chapter 6 Technique #2: Closeness Circle), and the media's perspective. Discuss how they impact the patient's life and appropriate weight.
- Promote self-care, including healthy exercise and diet. (See Chapter 3 Technique #1: Self-care.)
- Work on self-esteem that includes more than appearance. (See Chapter 3 Technique #12: Self-Esteem.)
- What are you grateful for about your body? (See Chapter 3 Technique #5: Happiness and Positives.)

Case #8.3: Since starting high school, her best friend is in a different class and has new friends. She is very upset about this and there have been negative interactions between them. The overwhelming negative emotions trigger a binge.

Question D: How do you help the patient identify triggers?

Discussion:

- Provide psychoeducation: See Chapter 9 Technique #3: Psychoeducation on Triggers.
- Use CBT:

Antecedent (Trigger)	Thoughts	Feelings	Body sensations	Behaviours
Seeing ex-best friend with her new friends	I'm not good enough to be her friend. The other girls are more attractive. She has abandoned me. Nobody likes me.	Angry, jealous, sad, lonely.	Craving for food. Flushed. Wanting to leave / move away from the situation.	Avoid negative feelings by bingeing.

- Connect life events (see Chapter 4 Technique #13: Variation A: Imagining a Timeline with Important Experiences) to fluctuation in eating disorder severity.

Question E: What can help with triggers?

Discussion:

- Teach Stage 1 Skills to help the patient stay in her window of tolerance (see Chapter 2 Technique #3: Window of Tolerance / Identify Intensity of Emotions), so she is not using bingeing to escape negative emotions. (See Chapter 9 Knowledge #10: Pathological Self-soothing / Addiction.)
- See Chapter 9 Technique #4: Working with Triggers.
- Use CBT: challenge the hot thoughts and find a balanced perspective. (See Chapter 5 Technique #16: Putting it Together.)
- Use IPT (see Chapter 6): teach skills to improve interpersonal interactions and build new relationships. Make the connection between the eating disorder and interpersonal difficulties.

Question F: What may be helpful to reduce bingeing?

Discussion:

- Plan regular healthy meals and snacks. This will help avoid hunger which may make the patient more vulnerable to bingeing. (See Technique #2: Addressing Vulnerabilities.)
- If the patient wants to binge, try plating only a portion of the food that she normally would have binged and putting the rest back in the fridge. After eating this smaller amount (which can reduce vulnerability), use a Stage 1 Skill or a distracting activity, then proceed mindfully.

- Use mindfulness: See Chapter 1 Technique #4: One Mindful Thing, and Chapter 7 Technique #22: Mindfulness of Craving.
- Use Chapter 7 Technique #2: STOP Skill.
- Address transition and interpersonal change. Grieve what is lost. (See Chapter 6 Technique #28: Grief.)

Case #8.4: After bingeing, she feels ashamed and compensates by restricting. She feels that she needs to be perfect and tries to keep her eating disorder a secret.

Question G: What can help reduce shame?

Discussion: See Chapter 7 Technique #8: Shame and Self-blame.

Question H: What can help address perfectionism?

Discussion:

- Teach self-compassion. (See Chapter 3 Technique #6: Self-Compassion.) Role-play a friend. (See Chapter 7 Technique #15: Role-playing Friend.)
- Challenge double standards of needing to be perfect while other people are not perfect. (See Chapter 5 Technique #1: Cognitive Distortions / Hot Thoughts.)

Case #8.5: The patient is much better at tolerating emotions after using Stage 1 Skills. She developed better self-esteem, one that is less tied to physical appearance and interactions with her ex-best friend. She plans regular healthy meals and snacks.

CASE #9: Teenager with Obsessive Compulsive Disorder (OCD)

Case #9.1: A sixteen-year-old female presenting with OCD. The patient is worried about contamination from toilets making her sick. She has excessive and prolonged handwashing and ritualized toileting routines. She tries to avoid public washrooms and this creates a problem for both school and social outings.

Question A: What screening tools can be used for OCD?

Discussion: Use Children's Yale-Brown Obsessive Compulsive Scale (CY-BOCS) for ages six to seventeen to screen for OCD, then use CY-BOCS Symptom Checklist to create a list of symptoms. For patients older than eighteen, use Yale-Brown Obsessive Compulsive Scale (Y-BOCS) and Y-BOCS Symptom Checklist.

Question B: How do you provide psychoeducation on obsession and compulsions?

Discussion: Thoughts, including intrusive thoughts, are normal products of the mind. It is the relationship to these thoughts (i.e., the appraisal of obsession and compulsion) and compulsive behaviours that keeps OCD alive. (See Chapter 5 Anxiety Model.)

Question C: What strategies can address obsessions?

Discussion:
- CBT:

Antecedent (Trigger)	Thoughts	Emotions and Intensity (0-100)	Body sensations
Toilets.	The toilet will contaminate me and I'll get sick and die.	Fear: 80. Anxiety: 90. Disgust: 90.	Heart beating fast. Chest tightness. Nausea.

Facts Supporting	Facts Against	Balanced Perspective	Re-rate Affect and Intensity
Toilet touches poop which has bacteria that can make people sick.	I have touched the toilet before and did not get sick. I have not died from a sickness. My body can fight off diseases.	Although the toilet has bacteria, my body can fight off diseases and I have not gotten sick or died from touching the toilet.	Fear: 40. Anxiety: 50. Disgust: 50.

- Use STOP Skill to tolerate distressing thoughts. (See Chapter 7 Technique #2: STOP Skill.)

Note: The therapist checks-in supportively, but not reassuringly. Help the patient self-reassure.

Question D: What strategies can address compulsion?

Discussion: Exposure treatment. (See Chapter 5 Techniques #19-22: Exposure Treatment.)

Case #9.2: The patient's goal is to be able to see her friends more often at school and at social gatherings, so she is motivated to overcome her fear of public toilets.

Question E: What strategies can help her reach her goal?

Discussion: Use ACT. (See Chapter 7 Technique #23: ACT.)

Note: Remind the patient of her motivation and agency.

Use mindfulness exercises to build acceptance of distressing thoughts.

Case #9.3: The patient successfully undergoes exposure therapy and was able to tolerate the distress of using public washrooms. She enjoys hanging out with her friends at the mall.

CASE #10: Hoarding

Case #10.1: A sixty-eight-year-old male presenting with hoarding. He lives alone in a crowded apartment. His sister is worried about him tripping over things and he is at risk of getting evicted due to the hoarding.

Question A: What are some complications of hoarding?

Discussion: Safety problems (falls, fire hazard), social conflicts, poor quality of life, functional impairments.

Question B: What strategies can help with hoarding?

Discussion:

- CBT: Challenge hot thoughts about acquiring / saving things and fear of throwing things away. (See Chapter 5 on CBT.)
- Make good social connections to reduce isolation. (See Chapter 6 on IPT.)
- Find other positive experiences (not just collecting things). (See Chapter 3 Fostering Positive Experiences.)
- Hire a professional organizer and cleaner to de-clutter.
- Use ACT to work towards the goal of living in a better environment. (See Chapter 7 Technique #23: ACT.)
- Bibliotherapy: Discuss the book *Buried in Treasures: Help for Compulsive Acquiring, Saving, and Hoarding* by David Tolin, Randy O. Frost, and Gail Steketee, either with the therapist or in a therapy group.

Case #10.2: The patient receives bibliotherapy in the form of group therapy and felt more connected to others during the therapy. He also did individual CBT to challenge hot thoughts about acquiring and saving things. His sister is very supportive throughout the process and they developed an even closer relationship. He also socializes more. He has a goal of living in a better environment, so when the interest rate dropped, he took the opportunity to purchase a home. His sister helped him rent a large garbage bin to clear out his apartment. He selected what he wanted to bring to his new home, so that it does not get cluttered. He resists the urge to purchase new things, so he keeps his new home uncluttered.

CASE #11: Substance Abuse

Case #11.1: An eighteen-year-old male presenting with substance abuse of OxyContin. He fractured his hand while playing competitive football two years ago. Due to complications of the injury, he could no longer play, which ruined his dream of getting into college by playing football. He felt the other player intentionally injured him to ruin his chance of college level football. He started using opioids after his hand surgery. Due to chronic pain, he was put on OxyContin. However, he has been taking more OxyContin than prescribed by purchasing from a dealer because his physician refused to increase the dose. He admits to taking OxyContin to help with stress and to "get a buzz."

Question A: What are the different stages of change and what could the therapist do for each stage?

Note: The medical management is beyond the scope of this book. Meet the patient at the stage they're at. Dr. James Prochaska et al. created the Transtheoretical Model of Behavior Change.

Discussion:

1) Precontemplative:
- Harm reduction e.g., What can you do to keep yourself safe when you use the substance?

- Increase patient's awareness of the problems e.g., What do you know about the substance?

2) Contemplative:
- Review pros and cons of treatment for addiction. (See Chapter 2 Technique #11: Pros and Cons.)
- Work with ambivalence. (See Chapter 5 Technique #17: Ambivalence / Working with Parts.)
- Increase patient motivation and confidence to change. (See Chapter 3 Technique #7: Values, and Technique #11: Mastery and Competence.)
    - E.g., What would make you feel ready for treatment?

3) Action:
- Set goals. (See Chapter 3 Technique #9: Setting Goals, and Chapter 8 Technique #5: Priorities and Align Goal / Getting Buy-in.)
- Work towards change. (See Chapter 5 Technique #15: Behaviour Activation.)

4) Maintenance:
- Prevent relapse. (Use Stage 1 Skills for coping.)

5) Relapse:
- Empower patients to restart contemplation and take action for their wellness.

Question B: How do you apply motivational interviewing?

Note: Dr. William Miller and Dr. Stephen Rollnick created Motivational interviewing in the 1980s.

Discussion:

Therapist: What made you want to come in today? (Start with open-ended questions.)

Patient: My life is a mess. I lost my job because I took too much OxyContin and worked too slowly. My mood is low and my pain is bothering me. My doctor won't give me any more pain meds. I got into a fight because I'm having difficulty affording more OxyContin from the dealer. I tried a cheaper pill and got really sick from it. I don't know what it was cut with. I'm getting into dangerous situations. I want to get my life together.

Therapist: Thank you for having the courage to share this and to get help. (Make affirmations.) When you say you want to get your life together, what would you like to work on? (Set goals.)

Patient: I want to feel better and have less pain without using as much OxyContin.

Therapist: On a scale of one to ten, ten being very important, how important is this goal? (Assess willingness to change.)

Patient: An eight.

Therapist: What makes you feel this way? (Explore motivation.)

Patient: I don't want to continue being unemployed and living in my parent's basement. I want to eventually go to college. I felt really scared after the fight and getting sick from the cheap pill. I don't want it to happen again.

Therapist: Sounds like you're really motivated to change. On a scale of one to ten, ten being immediate, when do you want to start working on your goal? (Explore readiness.)

Patient: A nine. I can't continue like this.

Therapist: (Nods.) How confident do you feel about being able to not take more OxyContin than prescribed, on a scale of one to ten, ten being very confident? (Explore ability to change.)

Patient: A two.

Therapist: What do you think is affecting your confidence?

Patient: I am worried that if I cut back on OxyContin my mood and pain would be worse. Also, if I fail at cutting back, I'll feel even worse about myself.

Therapist: Let me quickly summarize to make sure I have heard you correctly. You feel ready and motivated to cut back on OxyContin. You want to keep yourself safe and eventually go to college. You are worried about worsening pain and mood if you cut back on it? Is this correct?

Patient: Yes.

Therapist: Other than using OxyContin, what do you do to cope with the pain and low mood?

Question C: What psychotherapy strategies could help with chronic pain?

Discussion:

Therapist: Can you recall being pain free?

Patient: Yes. (If the patient says no and they've always had the pain, really question that.)

Therapist: What was going on in your life during that time?

Patient: I was practicing football and hoping to go to college on a scholarship for playing football. I was happy and life was good until I broke my hand.

Therapist: How do you feel now?

Patient: I feel angry and cheated about what happened. Now I'm stressed about what to do with my life instead. (If the patient has difficulty talking about emotions, teach language for emotions. See Chapter 2 Technique #1.)

Therapist: Pain and mood affect each other. Do you notice that your pain is worse when you feel more angry, cheated, anxious, or upset? (See Chapter 10 Case #7.2 regarding the mind-body connection and improving mood to improve pain.)

Patient: Yes.

Therapist: How bad is the pain on a scale of one to ten, ten being the worst possible pain?

Patient: Seven.

Therapist: Let's try using imagination to shrink negative emotions. (Do Chapter 4 Technique #4: Technique #7: Shrinking Negative Emotions. Then re-rate the pain intensity on a scale of one to ten.)

- See Chapter 4 Technique #4: Chronic Pain Management Techniques.
- See if pain improves by processing negative emotions or doing relaxation exercises. (See Chapter 7 Techniques #4-9 and Stage 1 Skills.)
- Imagine a mildly stressful stimulus on your left side. Try turning away from it and noticing how your body feels and whether there are any changes in pain sensation. (See Chapter 9 Technique #6: Working with Flight.)

Question D: What psychotherapy strategies could help with poor mood?

Discussion: See Stage 1 Skills.

Case #11.2: The patient used techniques from Chapter 4 to improve his chronic pain. Stage 1 Skills helped him better regulate his emotions. However, sometimes he still gets cravings.

Question E: What psychotherapy strategies could help with addressing cravings?

Discussion:

- Chapter 7 Technique #22: Mindfulness of Craving.
- Use Chapter 7 Technique #2: STOP Skill.
- Help the patient feel positive emotions rather than using OxyContin to "get a buzz." (See Chapter 3: Fostering Positive Experiences.)

Question F: What unprocessed loss (or trauma) may be present and fueling the addiction?

Discussion: Patient's hand injury and loss of the dream of playing college level football.

Question G: What psychotherapy strategies could help with addressing this loss?

Discussion:
- Narrative Exposure about his hand injury. (See Chapter 7 Techniques #17-21.)
- Grieve the loss of his dream. (See Chapter 6 Technique #28: Grief.)

Case #11.3: The patient processed the traumatic loss around his hand injury and grieved the loss of his dream of playing college football. Instead of escaping from his past using addiction, he can now face what happened. He goes jogging for exercise now and enjoys it. He is able to abstain from OxyContin and was able to find and keep another job.

Dysregulated Self and Relationship

CASE #12: Borderline Personality Disorder

Case #12.1: A twenty-year-old female with a diagnosis of BPD presenting with labile mood, interpersonal difficulties, and she self-harms by cutting. She has terminated relationships with two other therapists before.

Question A: How does hearing about this case make you feel? What thoughts are going through your mind?

Discussion: Sometimes therapists can feel concerned, anxious, and get a "heart sinking" feeling just from hearing about the patient. It is important to be aware of your own reactions and biases as this can affect the therapeutic relationship. The therapist needs to mentalize. (See Chapter 8 Knowledge #6: Step 1: Therapist Mentalizing.) Having positive feelings towards the patient and hoping that the patient could improve helps with the relationship and working towards treatment goals.

Question B: How would you approach this case?

Discussion: Work on building a strong therapeutic relationship first. Be clear about expectations and firm with boundaries. (See Chapter 8 Technique #2: Setting Expectations, and Technique #7: Maintaining Boundaries.) If the therapist is working on an interdisciplinary team or the patient sees multiple providers, be clear about each team member's role and have a united front. Sometimes the patient will create conflict amongst team members or split the team members into "good" people versus "bad" people.

It may be helpful to explore what happened with the other two therapists to see what could be done differently. Help the patient learn that relationships can be repaired. Explore the patient's fears about the therapeutic relationship and plan ahead. (See Chapter 8 Technique #18: Exploring Fears About the Relationship.) Emphasize that treatment requires collaboration and align treatment goals. (See Chapter 8 Technique #5: Priorities and Align Goal / Getting Buy-in.)

Question C: How may understanding attachment disorder help with the treatment of BPD?

Discussion: BPD is linked with insecure attachment. By treating attachment disorder, the patient's BPD symptoms could improve. The Healing the Inner Child technique could treat attachment disorder. (See Chapter 4 Technique #9.)

Question D: What psychotherapy strategies could help with labile mood?

Discussion: See Stage 1 Skills.

Question E: How could you address the cutting?

Discussion: The cutting is a pathological self-soothing behaviour. (See Chapter 9 Knowledge #10: Pathological Self-soothing / Addiction.) Assess the patient's readiness for change and use motivational interviewing skills. (See Chapter 10 Case #11.) For harm reduction, some patients find crushing ice can be helpful because it produces pain but does not come with the complications of cutting.

- Explore what cutting does for the patient. (See Chapter 2 Technique #9: Reflecting on Behaviour.)
- Identify and deal with triggers that lead to cutting. (See Chapter 9, Technique #4: Working with Triggers.) Use Stage 1 Skills to work with the intense emotions that the patient is coping with by cutting themselves.
- Self-hatred may contribute to cutting, so teach self-compassion. (See Chapter 3 Technique #6: Self-Compassion.)

Case #12.2: During one of the sessions, the patient started yelling at the therapist.

Question F: What can the therapist do?

Discussion:

- Use de-escalation skills. (See Chapter 6 Technique #17: De-escalation Skills.) Then do a Stage 1 Skill together.
- Patients with BPD are relationally challenged with both the therapist and others, so teach interpersonal skills. (See Chapter 6.) They tend to have a narrow window of tolerance, so they may quickly use a defence response. Address the defence responses. (See Chapter 9 Techniques #5-10.)
- Validate the patient, then challenge them to improve. (See Chapter 8 Technique #13: Balancing between Validation and Challenge.)

- Reinforce boundaries and expectations. The therapist can bring up the contract, supporting that therapy needs to be safe for both people. (See Chapter 8 Technique #3: Sample Contract.)
- Address traumatic re-enactments. (See Chapter 8 Knowledges #6-8 and Techniques #20-24.)

Case #12.3: She uses Stage 1 Skills to help her move back into her window of tolerance. Instead of cutting, she either crushes ice or applies a Stage 1 Skill. Gradually, she develops a strong therapeutic relationship with her therapist. By addressing traumatic re-enactments, the therapist is able to repair the relationship. The patient learns that relationships can be repaired and develops strategies to improve her interpersonal relationships. Between using the Healing the Inner Child technique and the therapeutic relationship, her attachment disorder is repaired. She is able to have more fulfilling interpersonal relationships.

PTSD / Simple Trauma

CASE #13: Acute Stress in a Refugee

Case #13.1: A forty-nine-year-old female presenting to a family physician's office as a new patient. She is a refugee who has recently left a war zone and appears very anxious at the physician's office.

Question A: What is psychological first aid (PFA)?

Note: National Child Traumatic Stress Network and the National Center for PTSD created PFA.

Discussion: PFA is a technique for patients who have had a recent traumatic event. It is used to decrease distress and improve coping and function.

Note: Not all survivors or refugees need treatment. Treat patients who are distressed, disoriented, or outside their window of tolerance. (See Chapter 2 Technique #3: Window of Tolerance.)

Question B: What are the goals of PFA?

Discussion:

- Address the patient's immediate needs and concerns.
- Use the therapeutic relationship to provide safety, calmness, and compassion.
- Support healthy coping strategies and empower patients to move toward recovery.
- Connect the patient to social networks and supports.

Question C: How do you provide PFA?

Discussion: See Chapter 8 Knowledge #5: Therapist Stance for Trauma-informed Care.

Note: If using an interpreter, look and speak to the patient that is being addressed and not the interpreter.

1) Calm

Therapist: You seem anxious. Let's do some breathing exercises together. (See Chapter 8 Technique #1: Slow Outbreath.) How are you feeling now?

2) Gather information

Therapist: How can I help you?

Patient: I don't know.

Therapist: Is there anything you are worried about?

Patient: I am currently in a shelter. I am worried about safety and how long I can stay there.

Therapist: (Explore immediate / basic needs including food, water, clothing, finances, housing, and medical care.)

3) Assist

Therapist: May I connect you with our social worker who can help you with your housing concern? (Connect patients to social services including childcare. Connect them socially: to find a community, spiritual support, or reunite with loved ones, family, and friends.)

Patient: Yes.

4) Provide psychoeducation about stress reactions.

Therapist: People who experience stressful events can feel numb or negative emotions, such as anger, sadness, and anxiety. They may experience physical symptoms of stress, such as heart palpitations, shortness of breath, and have sleep problems. People may try to avoid reminders of the stressful event. What are some coping strategies that you use when you are stressed?

5) Coping Skills
- Address pathological coping strategies including connecting the patient to addiction services. (See Chapter 9 Knowledge #10: Pathological Self-soothing and Addiction.)
- Highlight their strengths and that they managed to keep themselves safe. (See Chapter 3 Technique #13: Fostering Hope and Optimism.)
- If they feel helpless, explore when they previously felt they had control.
- Teach them how to work with triggers. (See Chapter 9 Technique #4: Working with Triggers.)
- Teach new coping strategies. (See Stage 1 Skills.)
- Encourage self-care and having a routine.

Case #13.2: The patient calmed down. She connected with a social worker who helped her find stable housing, connect with her relatives, and join a community of people from similar cultural backgrounds. She did not develop PTSD. She is also taking free English classes and is settling into her new life and routine.

CASE #14: Dog Attack

Case #14.1: An eight-year-old male presenting with PTSD after being attacked by his neighbour's dog. He has some scarring on his right arm, but otherwise is physically well. However, psychologically, he has become very anxious and avoids playing outside. This is interfering with his ability to socialize. He has also developed nightmares and sometimes tries to avoid going to bed. The dog was euthanized, and he feels guilty about this. His mother feels he is more disruptive at home than he was previously, but she is worried and feels guilty about disciplining him given the traumatic event.

Question A: How do you provide psychoeducation?

Discussion:

Therapist: When a child experiences trauma, anxiety, avoidance, and nightmares can develop as part of PTSD. In addition to typical PTSD symptoms, children can also become more disruptive, defiant, and aggressive after trauma. (See Chapter 9 Knowledge #7: PTSD, and Technique #2: Psychoeducation.)

Question B: What parenting strategies may be helpful?

Discussion:

- Use praise effectively for desired behaviours. Consistently praise the specific behaviour immediately when it occurs. Avoid mixed messaging, i.e. do not add negative messages to the praise, and make sure the tone is congruent with the praise.
    - E.g., "Great job putting the dishes into the sink after dinner!"

- NOT: "Good." (Too vague). "Good job on winning the regional competition, but why have you never won at the provincial level?" (Mixed messaging).
- Use active ignoring for undesirable and not dangerous behaviour. Do not ignore unsafe behaviours. Ignore undesired verbal communication to the parent such as mocking, angry copying, or defiant statements. Ignore undesired non-verbal communication to the parent such as eye-rolling or making ugly faces. Avoid both verbal and non-verbal communication (e.g., eye contact) with the child during and immediately after the undesired behaviour.
- Combine active ignoring with effective praise. Praise the child for accepting no. E.g., "Thank you for putting your toys away and coming for dinner. You're so well behaved!"
- Use time-outs for discipline (for children less than age eleven or twelve). Do not use ineffective strategies such as yelling or hitting a child as this may instead model undesired behaviour. Time-out length: Using one minute times the age of the child is generally a good length, but there's no hard rule. Be consistent. Pick a quiet place for time-outs.
  - E.g., "Do not throw toys. I am giving you a warning. If you do that again, I will put you in a time-out." Then the child throws another toy. "I am putting you in a time-out because you threw another toy after I told you to stop. You are going to stay in the time-out for eight minutes to think about your behaviour." Put the child in a time-out and set the timer. Use active ignoring for the duration of the time-out, except for unsafe behaviour or escaping. If the child escapes, put them back in

the time-out with minimal communication (avoid speaking / eye contact) and reset the timer. Repeat this until the child stays in the time-out for the entire duration. At the end of time-out, restate why it happened and get an apology. "You are in a time-out because I asked you to stop throwing toys and you threw another toy. You need to apologize to me for not listening." "Sorry mom." "Thank you for apologizing. Now, give me a hug."
- Model desired behaviour.
- Use a behaviour chart. Pick one behaviour to work on at a time. Talk to the child about how to get stars and decide together about rewards. Tally up the stars for rewards daily or weekly (daily for younger children). Be consistent.
- Practice parenting strategies with the parent. (See Chapter 6 Technique #26: Therapist Role-playing.)

Note: The word parent is used, but this can be a guardian, or any supportive adult in the child's life.

Case #14.2: The mother is no longer worried about discipline and uses time-outs as discipline. By using active ignoring with effective praise and a behaviour chart, the child's behaviour improves. However, he experiences ongoing anxiety and still avoids playing outside.

Question C: What psychotherapy strategies may be helpful for anxiety and avoidance?

Note: Trauma-Focused Cognitive Behavior Therapy (TF-CBT) was developed by Dr. Anthony Mannarino et al. for use with children and adolescents.

Discussion:
- Teach language for emotions. (See Chapter 2 Technique #1.)

- Use relaxation techniques. (See Chapter 10 Case #5: Child with Anxiety.)
- Use CBT to challenge hot thoughts. (See Chapter 5.)
- Use narrative exposure. (See Chapter 7 Techniques #17-21.)
- Use hypnotic techniques to work with the traumatic memory. The patient may want to imagine being around dogs before real-life exposure. (See Chapter 6 Techniques #14-16: Working with Traumatic Memories.)
- Expose the patient to dogs and go outside. (See Chapter 5 Techniques #19-22: Exposure Treatment.)
- Help the child share the trauma narrative with the parent. Then co-create safety plans (E.g., how to stay safe in the neighbourhood).

Note: Other treatments that can be helpful for PTSD are EMDR and neurofeedback. They are beyond the scope of this book.

Question D: What strategies can address the patient's guilt?

Discussion: See Chapter 7 Technique #7: Guilt.

By using Chapter 5 Technique #9: Assigning Responsibility, he feels less guilty, because he believes both the dog and its owner have responsibility about the dog bite and the dog getting euthanized.

Note: The parent may also need separate psychotherapy treatment.

Question E: What strategies can address nightmares?

Discussion:

- Use redreaming technique. (See Chapter 4 Technique #11: Working with Nightmares.)
- Boost self-esteem at bedtime, which helps create positive feelings and belief that one has the coping skills. (See Chapter 3 Technique #12: Self-Esteem.)

- If the patient wakes up in the middle of the night from a nightmare, do a grounding exercise to get oriented to the present. (See Chapter 1 Technique #2: Orienting to the Present, and Technique #3: Engaging the Five Senses.) Don't think about the meaning of the nightmare as this may worsen the sleep / nightmares.
- Address sleep avoidance. Sleep deprivation increases the number of dreams.
- If the patient fears not being able to wake up if there is danger, reassure them that well-rested people wake up more easily and with better judgment and less confusion.
- Avoid checking for safety at bed time as this may worsen anxiety and instead use the opposite action. (See Chapter 7 Technique #3: Opposite Action.)

Case #14.3: The patient is able to calm down using relaxation techniques. His guilt is significantly reduced and he no longer gets nightmares. He successfully underwent exposure treatment and is able to play outside and be around dogs again.

Dissociation

CASE #15: Dissociation and Peripartum Mental Health

Case #15.1: A thirty-four-year-old female presented to her family physician in the first trimester of her pregnancy, which is uncomplicated. This is a planned pregnancy and her husband is overjoyed. Her husband is wondering if she is depressed. She thought she would feel happy, but she doesn't. She does not feel sad. She just feels numb, but she feels this is normal for her. She is wondering if this is a problem. She is still working a busy job with long hours. Sometimes when it gets really busy, she notices that her body feels unreal, she feels outside of her body, the environment feels foggy, or things feel further away.

Question A: Are the symptoms that the patient describes concerning?

Discussion: The patient is describing the symptoms of dissociation: emotional numbing, depersonalization (her body feels unreal and she feels outside of her body), and derealization (the environment feels foggy or things feel further away.) (See Chapter 9 Knowledge #11: Dissociation.)

Question B: What tool can screen for dissociative disorders?

Discussion: Dissociative Experiences Scale (DES-II).

Case #15.2: The patient's DES-II score is twenty-seven. She has been having dissociative experiences since she was about eight years old. From ages eight to ten she had a step-father who emotionally and physically abused her. Her mother, who was a single mom, aside from this two year period, relies on the patient for support. She felt that she had to keep it together for her mother, so she has never addressed the abuse. She is open to treatment.

Question C: What strategies may help her dissociation?

Discussion:

- Provide psychoeducation about dissociation and help the patient commit to treating dissociation. Explore the pros and cons of dissociation, which is a pathological coping strategy. (See Chapter 2 Technique #11: Pros and Cons.)
- Use mindfulness and body techniques to help her be present and stay connected to her body. (See Chapter 1 Stage 1 Skills, especially Technique #2: Orienting to the Present, Technique #3: Engaging the Five Senses, Technique #6: Mindful Movements, Technique #10: Grounding on Uneven Grounds, and Technique #11: Dual Awareness with Hands.)

- Teach about emotions including myths. (See Chapter 2 Technique #2: Addressing Fears and Myths about Emotions.)
- When dissociated, the patient cannot feel negative emotions, but also cannot feel positive emotions. Help her feel both positive and negative emotions. (See Chapter 2 Techniques #1-2, and Chapter 3 Fostering Positive Experiences.) Treat emotional numbing early on as patients need to feel, to process and heal from the trauma.
- Help her tolerate emotions using Stage 1 Skills. Patients with dissociation tend to be more hypnotizable, so hypnotic techniques tend to work well. Play to their strengths. (See Chapter 4.)
- Explore what makes her more likely to dissociate. (See Chapter 3 Technique #2: Addressing Vulnerabilities.) Address the triggers, including work stress as a trigger. (See Chapter 9 Technique #4: Working with Triggers.)
- Sometimes patients use dissociation when it is difficult to accept reality, so using Chapter 7 Technique #1: Radical Acceptance to accept reality may reduce dissociation.
- Identify early symptoms / signs of dissociation. What do they notice right before the dissociative experience? What do they feel in their body? Are there any thoughts that preceded the experience? (E.g., This is unreal. I can't take this.)
- Teach strategies to work with the faint response. (See Chapter 9 Technique #8: Working with Faint.)

Case #15.3: She now notices when she starts to dissociate and uses Stage 1 Skills to bring herself back to her window of tolerance. She is now able to experience both positive and negative emotions. She understands emotions are transient and better tolerates them. She finds that her emotions help her connect better with her husband and emotions are helpful rather than a hindrance. She notices that at work, she has to try harder to not dissociate. She has never asked for a reduced workload. She's wondering if she should, but she also feels that she enjoys keeping busy.

Question D: How would you address her question about her work?

Discussion: Sometimes patients use workaholism to avoid processing traumatic memories. (See Chapter 9 Knowledge #10 Pathological Self-soothing / Addiction.) Trauma often affects self-esteem, and workaholism sometimes is used to boost self-esteem. Help the patient find healthy ways to boost self-esteem. (See Chapter 3 Technique #12: Self-Esteem.) Sometimes when people feel unwanted (in childhood), they may try to make themselves feel needed.

Narrating the abusive experiences in a self-compassionate way may also help with self-esteem as sometimes patients blame themselves for what happened. (See Chapter 7 Technique #17: Narrative Exposure, and Chapter 9 Technique #8: Shame and Self-blame.)

Patients with dissociation are at risk of further traumatization, because they have trouble standing up for themselves. Help the patient try to be safe, as being unsafe leads to more dissociation. The patient may need to learn to say no to people. (See Chapter 3 Technique #8: Setting Boundaries.) Ultimately, it is the patient's choice how much work she wants to do. (See Chapter 8 Technique #10: Choice.) Help the patient have a balanced perspective and foster problem solving. (See Chapter 3 Technique #10: Problem Solving.) Moreover, help her improve interpersonal relationships, have healthier interpersonal interactions and more supportive people in her life. (See Chapter 6 IPT.)

Note: Pregnancy can be a powerful motivator for patients to seek treatment and improve.

Case #15.4: She understands that she was using workaholism to both boost her self-esteem and to avoid the trauma memories. She develops a healthier sense of self. She is better at setting boundaries and decides to cut back on work, so she can take better care of herself. She was able to tolerate and process her trauma memory in a self-compassionate way and grieve what she missed in her childhood. Although she cannot change her childhood, she can give her child what she would have liked to have in her childhood. She is much happier and feels excited, albeit a bit anxious, about becoming a mom.

Complex Trauma

CASE #16: Complex PTSD in a Veteran

Case #16.1: A fifty-seven-year-old male veteran presenting with PTSD, substance abuse with alcohol and opioids, and mixed personality disorder traits (Cluster B and C traits.) He is a smoker, has diabetes, peripheral vascular disease (PVD) with bilateral below knee amputations, and chronic pain post amputation. He complains of poor sleep, low mood, and pain, and they adversely affect each other.

Question A: What in the clinical presentation makes you suspect complex PTSD rather than simple PTSD?

Discussion: The patient has multiple psychiatric and medical diagnoses. He has issues with mood, dysregulated physiology (sleep disorder), addictive behaviours, chronic pain, and relational issues (personality disorders). He is also sicker than an average person his age. (See Chapter 9 Knowledge #14: When to Consider DTD and CT.)

Note: In a patient with complex PTSD, screen for dissociation.

Question B: Using the Stepwise Treatment, how would you organize your approach to treatment?

Discussion: Stabilize the patient first before processing the traumatic memories. (See Chapter 9 Knowledge #16: Step 1 Stabilizing.)
- Help patients feel safe and establish rapport.
- Provide psychoeducation about trauma and its impact. (See Chapter 9 Technique #2: Psychoeducation.)
- Help patients stay calm and regulate their emotions. (See Stage 1 Skills.)

Question C: How might understanding attachment help with the treatment of cPTSD?

Discussion: Complex trauma usually involves invasive and interpersonal trauma. Therefore, he likely has insecure attachment. Treating attachment disorder early on can improve interpersonal relationships, which can improve the therapeutic relationship. Chapter 4 Technique #9: Healing the Inner Child could treat attachment disorder, and also improve mood, self-esteem, and sleep.

Question D: How would you motivate the patient towards change?

Discussion: Align goals and use the patient's goal to motivate him to engage in healthy behaviour. Alcohol and opioids can worsen sleep, so explore whether the patient is open to addressing addiction. Medical health impacts mental health, so explore the patient's readiness to work on his physical health. (See Chapter 8 Technique #5: Priorities and Align Goal / Getting Buy-in.)

Note: Try to have the patient optimized medically. Poorly controlled PVD can cause pain, and poorly controlled diabetes increases risk of developing depression.

Case #16.2: The patient is motivated by wanting to improve his sleep, mood, and pain. He is willing to work with the therapist.

By doing Stage 1 Skills together, the therapist builds rapport with the patient and the patient is able to feel calmer and more safe. Through both the Healing the Inner Child technique and the therapeutic relationship, the patient's attachment disorder improves. He no longer meets diagnostic criteria for a personality disorder. His mood improves and he understands how his mood affects his physical symptoms. His sleep and pain also improves a bit. He's interested in additional strategies to improve sleep and pain.

Question E: What strategies may help with sleep?

Discussion:

- Using pillows for positioning to lessen pain may also improve sleep.
- Work with insomnia and nightmares. (See Chapter 10 Case #6: Senior with Insomnia, and Case #14: Dog Attack.)

Question F: What psychotherapy strategies may help with pain?

Discussion: See Chapter 10 Case #11: Substance abuse, Question C.

Case #16.3: His mood, sleep, and pain issues are much better controlled. He is working with the physician to reduce opioids, smoking, and alcohol. He understands that unresolved trauma is affecting both his mental and physical health and he is motivated to treat this. He starts talking about his past in greater detail. He has a history of childhood emotional and physical abuse from his parents. He joined the military at age sixteen to escape the family situation, but was further traumatized by witnessing comrades get injured and die in combat. He left the military in his early thirties due to mental illness.

Question G: How do you know when the patient is ready to process the trauma memory?

Discussion: Although trauma recovery is broken into three steps, in reality, this is not a linear process, and the patient goes back and forth between the steps. It is helpful to practice the Stage 1 Skills, so that the patient has emotional regulation skills. Some patients may jump into sharing trauma stories right away. It is important for the patient to stay grounded while discussing the trauma memory, so they are not reliving the experience. If the patient is not able to stay grounded and tolerate the emotions, slow down. (See Chapter 7 Technique #18: Staying Grounded while Processing Traumatic Memory and Chapter 8 Technique #9: Slowing Down the Process.)

Some patients may choose not to talk about the trauma memory at this point in time. It is important to respect the patient's choice. Patients whose avoidance of the trauma memory is causing problems such as having flashbacks, nightmares, or using pathological self-soothing to suppress the memories, will likely benefit from exploring the trauma memory. Use ambivalence and motivational interviewing to help the patient move towards change. (See Chapter 5 Technique #17: Ambivalence / Working with Parts, and Chapter 10 Case #11: Substance Abuse, Question A.)

Question H: What strategies can help the patient process the trauma memory?

Discussion:

- See Chapter 9 Knowledge #17: Step 2 Processing Memory.
- See Chapter 1 Technique #18: Mindful Action with Traumatic Memory.
- See Chapter 3 Stage 2 Skills, Technique #18: Rewriting Your Story and Reframing, Technique #19: Self-Forgiveness, and Technique #20: Forgiving Others.
- Help the patient grieve the loss of childhood, innocence, hope, dreams, purpose, illusion of safety and

predictability, and the old-self. (See Chapter 4 Technique #12: Funeral of the Broken Dreams, and Chapter 6 Technique #28: Grief.)
- See Chapter 4 Technique #13: Variation A: Imagining a Timeline with Important Experiences and Working with Traumatic Memories Techniques #14-16.
- See Chapter 4 Techniques #19-22: Exposure Treatment.
- See Chapter 7 Stage 2 Skills Techniques #4-23: Changing Trauma-related Emotions, Beliefs and Behaviours.

Case #16.4: By going back and forth between processing trauma memory and Stage 1 Skills, he's able to tolerate and consolidate the trauma. He can reflect on his past with self-compassion. He grieves the loss of his childhood and his fallen comrades. His PTSD symptoms, including nightmares and flashbacks are resolved. He is able to tolerate both positive and negative emotions by using Stage 1 Skills. He successfully quits alcohol and smoking. His pain is well controlled with only non-opioid medications.

Question I: What would be a good point to discharge the patient?

Discussion:
- See Chapter 9 Knowledge #18: Step 3 Post-traumatic Growth / New Normal.
- Generally therapy reduces suffering and improves function and can be terminated when treatment goals are met. There's no firm rules on when to discharge the patient, but involve the patient in the discussion, including what the next steps are. Some patients may return later for "booster" sessions.
- Given that the patient is bothered by his sleep, mood, and pain, treatment goals include improved sleep, being able to regulate emotions and feel pleasure (without pathological self-soothing), and better pain control.
- Resolve / reduce PTSD symptoms.

- Have good coping skills rather than addiction.
- Improve interpersonal function and better social support.
- Improve self-care, which includes better chronic disease management (better control of diabetes and PVD).
- Improved self-esteem and more self-compassion.
- Finding meaning and purpose: figuring out what it means to live well and what he can still do despite limitations (i.e. despite having bilateral below knee amputations and other medical conditions).
- Leave the patient with hope and optimism for the future. (See Chapter 3 Technique #13: Fostering Hope and Optimism.)

Case #16.5: He takes much greater care of his physical health, including doing upper body exercises and eating healthy. As a result, his diabetes and PVD are much better controlled. He makes a new friend who enjoys woodworking and invites him to do it together. He now enjoys making wooden toys as a hobby and finds meaning in donating them to children in need. The therapist and patient agreed to terminate therapy. The patient knows how to reconnect with the therapist if he feels the need for booster sessions, but he feels optimistic that he has the strategies and social support to cope with new life challenges.

CASE #17: Dissociative Identity Disorder (DID)

Case #17.1: A twenty-two-year-old female university student presenting with both PTSD and severe dissociative symptoms. She was doing well academically until she was physically assaulted by a stranger on the subway. She felt like the assault had "thrown her off the cliff" from a mental health perspective. Her DES-II score is forty-eight.

Question A: What tools are helpful for diagnosis of DID?

Discussion:
- Use the DES-II and ask the patient for more details about any of the experiences they have for at least twenty percent of the time.
- Other tools: Multidimensional Inventory of Dissociation (MID), Dissociative Disorders Interview Schedule (DDIS), Structured Clinical Interview for DSM-IV Dissociative Disorders, Revised (SCID-D-R).

Case #17.2: Prior to the assault, she frequently felt numb and had very poor memories of her childhood. She hears and sees the "other internal people" in her "mind's eyes and ears." Since the assault, she has been having nightmares and flashbacks, including some "forgotten" memories of her childhood which have come back and are haunting her. She intermittently "blanks out." She believes that when she "blanks out," one of the internal people takes over, so she doesn't know what happened during this period. All of these are interfering with her academic performance.

Question B: How would you organize your approach to treatment?

Discussion: (See Chapter 9 Stepwise Treatment Knowledge #16-18.)

Step 1: Stabilizing:
- See Chapter 10 Case #16 Question B.
- Help the patient re-integrate identity / self. (See Question D below.)

Step 2: Processing Memory: Re-integrate parts of the traumatic memory, such as emotions, bodily sensations, thoughts, and behaviour. Then re-integrate traumatic memory with non-traumatic memory to form a cohesive self-narrative.

Step 3: Post-traumatic Growth / New Normal.

Question C: What are some possible functions of alters or "internal people?"

Discussion:

Therapist: How have the alters helped you? (See Chapter 3 Technique #4: Reframing.)
- Protect the patient from unbearable feelings or memories.
- Distance the patient from responsibility: "The alters did this."
- Distance the patient from reality: "This happened to the alters." (Some patients have non-human alters to distance themselves from the cruelty of mankind.)
- Address intense mixed feelings or conflicting beliefs by seeing this as coming from different "internal people."
- Compartmentalize the trauma so that the patient can continue to live a "normal life."
- To hide information from themselves (e.g., keep money hidden from themselves).
- To hide unacceptable behaviours (e.g., the patient's parents were against her creating art, so one of her alters creates art without her knowing.)
- Mentally escape an unbearable or inescapable situation by "blanking out."
- Helps them to maintain relationships with the abuser (address attachment needs.)
- Address loneliness and have relationships with the alter.
- Act as a shortcut to help the patient behave certain ways in certain situations or around certain people. (E.g., A female patient could have a male identifying alter to help her carry out what are traditionally male roles.)

Question D: What strategies can help reintegrate the alters back into the self?

Discussion:
- Use Chapter 4 Technique #9: Healing the Inner Child, or Variation A: Imagining Ideal Parents. Each alter may need a different ideal parent figure. This provides a safe space

for the alters to come out. When they come out, leave them out.
- Therapist: When you come for therapy, you and all of your alters must be present. When they come out, leave them out. Practice leaving them all out all the time.
- Therapist: Imagine a group meeting with all your alters in a safe place. Get to know them. (See Chapter 4 Technique #1: Imagining a Safe Place.)
- Therapist: Imagine stepping into an alter and blending with them. Imagine blending all your alters together.
- The therapist needs to be consistent, treating all the alters as the same person rather than as separate people. Do not pick favourites between alters. Be aware of traumatic re-enactments, such as the therapist trying to be the rescuer when an adult patient's child-like alter comes out. (See Chapter 8 Addressing Traumatic Re-enactment, Knowledges #7-9.)
- Use radical acceptance: The patient accepts that what happened to the alters happened to them. What the alters did, they did, because alters are aspects of self. Process the grief associated with this.
- Prevent "blanking out" or switching out to an alter by paying attention to awareness. (See Chapter 1 Technique #17: Combine Mindfulness about Absentmindedness and Mindfulness about being Present.)
- Therapist to identify when the patient is "switching" and help the patient ground themselves. If the patient is giving inaccurate information, for example an adult patient believing that they are a child, challenge this and help the patient ground by using the five senses and looking at themselves.
- Do pros and cons of having alters. Problem solve through this. (E.g., Instead of "blanking out" to escape painful

emotions, use Chapter 4 Technique #6: Auto-hypnosis using a Mirror.)
- Help the patient work through conflict between alters. (See Chapter 5 Technique #17: Ambivalence / Working with Parts.) Traumatic re-enactments can also occur between alters. (See Chapter 8 Knowledge #3: Traumatic Re-enactment.)
- Reduce dissociation in general. (See Chapter 10 Case #15 Question C for strategies to reduce dissociation.)
- Help the patient connect with reality and distinguish between reality versus internal thoughts and feelings. Use grounding techniques and cognitive dissonance to challenge the patient when they are struggling with reality and not making sense. (E.g., Therapist: "Help me make sense of this. You believe you are five years old, but if you look in a mirror, you notice that you are in an adult's body.")

Case #17.3: The patient notices when she starts dissociating and gets herself back to the window of tolerance using Stage 1 Skills. She understands the "other internal people" are all aspects of herself and now knows all of them. She notices that previously she dreamed about the alters as separate people, but now she has dreams about herself as one person. She has a much better integrated sense of self and no longer "blanks out." There are no safety concerns. She is still bothered by nightmares and flashbacks. The traumatic memories come back to her in pieces, such as a scream, taste of blood in her mouth, and images.

Question E: What can be done next?

Note: Sometimes flashbacks can be somatic only (e.g., taste of blood) or emotion only, i.e., no narrative.

Discussion: Given the patient is stabilized and has a more integrated sense of self, proceed with Steps 2. (See Chapter 10 Case #16 Question H.)

Try to figure out the original traumatic memories from flashbacks. Connect the somatic sensation and feelings with the original trauma. CBT can be used to process the feelings and thoughts that come up. (See Chapter 7 Techniques #4-21.) Patients with dissociation have the tendency to go numb, so check in during processing of traumatic memory to make sure that the patient can still feel. If they are not able to feel emotions, they are not processing the trauma memory. Return to Stage 1 Skills as needed to stay in the window of tolerance and get out of dissociation. Once the patient has mastery over these "natural" exposures and can stay present, move onto more recall of trauma memory. If alters are still present, get permission from all of them to go into the trauma memory before proceeding. Acceptance and recall of trauma memory will help with the fusion of alters. Communicate with other alters to get trauma memories.

Case #17.4: The patient's nightmares and flashbacks have resolved. She now has cohesive memories of childhood abuse and confronted her father about this. Her father responded by saying that it was not child abuse, but rather normal punishment because she was a bad kid. Her father has not hurt her physically as an adult, but continues to be emotionally abusive. She finds that she goes numb when having to deal with him.

Question F: What are common strategies used by the perpetrator?

Discussion: The perpetrator normalizes or trivializes the abusive behaviours and blames or undermines the victim.

Question G: What strategies may help the patient?
Discussion:

- Given that the patient still has ongoing attachment with the perpetrator, help the patient try to stay safe. Being unsafe leads to more dissociation.
- Help the patient notice their stress and use Stage 1 Skills to calm down and stay grounded.

- Help her be aware of her emotions and validate her feelings. Teach the patient to use healthy strategies to express her emotions rather than numbing them (E.g., Labelling her emotions, journaling, and creating art).
- Explore with the patient "What is going on? What do I need right now? How can I address my needs?
- Teach the patient to say no and set boundaries. (See Chapter 3 Technique #8: Setting Boundaries.)
- Improve the patient's interpersonal skills to see if the relationship can be improved. (See Chapter 6.) If the relationship cannot be improved, sometimes the patient needs to grieve and move on.

Case #17.5: The patient realizes that her father is not ready to take responsibility for what happened or to change. She sets boundaries with him and limits their contact. Instead, she now spends a lot more time with supportive friends from the university. Her academic performance is now back on track.

Special Populations

The techniques covered in this book can generally be applied to school age children all the way up to patients with mild dementia.

For infant and preschool children: Attachment issues are a big concern. Help the parents acquire better parenting skills and get treatment for their own mental illness and attachment disorder. (See Case #14.)

For patients with advanced dementia or those who cannot tolerate the traditional one-to-one talk therapy, consider pet therapy, music therapy, or recreational therapy (which is equivalent to play therapy for children).

Therapist Wellness and Peak Performance

Question A: Why is it important for the therapist to take care of themselves?

Discussion: Healing occurs in the therapeutic relationship. The therapist needs to be well and be aware of their own state of mind, so they can co-regulate with the patient and provide a safe environment for healing.

Question B: What strategies can help with therapist wellness?

Discussion:

- Engage in healthy practices: (See Chapter 3 Technique #1: Self-care) and find five minutes a day to apply the Stage 1 Skills for themselves.
- Get treatment early (i.e., therapists / doctors for therapists). Sometimes therapists are reluctant to seek help due to fear of stigma, discrimination, and licensing concerns. Being well helps the therapist function optimally, which then improves patient care.
- Be mindful of your own needs and limitations.
- Find supportive people. Join a peer supervision group or a buddy system (where the therapist checks in with themselves to make sure they are alright, and checks in with two other therapists to make sure they are also alright).
- Maintain healthy boundaries and do not overwork. (See Chapter 3 Technique #8: Setting Boundaries.)
- Have a sense of self-agency. (See Chapter 3 Technique #15: Building Resilience.)
- Develop a reflective practice such as journaling. (See Chapter 2 Technique #12: Journaling.)

Question C: What strategies can help with peak performance?

Discussion:
- Be in the window of tolerance. (See Chapter 2 Technique #3: Window of Tolerance.)
- Use a Stage 1 Skill such as the STOP Skill when outside the window of tolerance. (See Chapter 7 Technique #2: STOP Skill.)
- Do one mindful thing at a time. Multitasking decreases efficiency because time is wasted switching between tasks rather than doing two things simultaneously. (E.g., Try doing math by subtracting twenty-seven from ninety-three while imagining drinking lemonade. Most people are switching between the tasks rather than doing both simultaneously.) (See Chapter 1 Technique #4: One Mindful Thing.)
- Be self-compassionate. This decreases anxiety and improves motivation. (See Chapter 3 Technique #6: Self-Compassion.)
- Set achievable goals and let go of perfectionism. (See Chapter 3 Technique #9: Setting Goals.)
- Have healthy self-esteem rather than one that is tied to achievements. (See Chapter 3 Technique #12: Self-Esteem.)
- Think about what you are grateful for. (See Chapter 3 Technique #5: Happiness and Positives.)
- Find meaning in the work you do. (See Chapter 3 Technique #14: Finding Meaning.)
- Have hope and optimism about your work and your patients. (See Chapter 3 Technique #13: Fostering Hope and Optimism.)
- Thank yourself for the wonderful work that you do.

Summary

Patients are resilient and can recover from many different traumas. They are also capable of learning new strategies. Patients with cognitive impairment can be treated with modified techniques or strategies other than traditional one-on-one talk therapy. There's no "one size fits all" treatment. Play to the patient's strengths and explore and try new strategies.

Identify and treat attachment disorders early on. Use the therapeutic relationship and Healing the Inner Child technique to do so. When treating patients with relational challenges, discuss the therapeutic relationship, address trauma re-enactments, and repair the relationship.

Pathological behaviours are behaviours that have previously been useful for coping, but are now causing problems. Working with ambivalence and motivational interviewing can help motivate patients to use new coping strategies instead of self-defeating behaviours. For patients with multiple diagnoses, it may be more helpful to organize the symptoms as dysregulated mood, physiology, attention, behaviour, self, and relationship.

This type of work is not easy, and it is important that therapists take care of themselves, so they can then take care of their patients.

CONCLUSION

Using the concept of behavioural activation and committing to practising techniques for five minutes a day, both patients and therapists can learn and improve themselves. Being trauma-informed is an universal stance that helps patients recover from mental illnesses.

The therapeutic relationship, and the connection it provides, is key to healing. Effective communication and collaboration with the patient helps them move towards their treatment goals. The therapist needs to create a calm and safe environment, by building trust, providing containment, being consistent, and upholding boundaries. Encouraging curiosity helps patients explore, while providing choices empowers them. Be mindful of cultural differences. Build on the patient's strengths, boost their coping skills, improve their competence and sense of mastery to build resilience and improve self-esteem. Lastly, help patients find hope and meaning in their lives.

With many techniques to choose from, this book empowers both patients and therapists to find what works for them. Mindfulness and body techniques help ground patients and can change physical symptoms and sensations. Mentalizing helps patients self-reflect and better understand themselves and the world. Fostering positive experiences and reframing help patients improve self-esteem, and create hope and meaning. Using imagination and hypnotic techniques create new possibilities, including new behaviours, thoughts, and feelings. CBT and its variations treat many different mental health issues. IPT can help improve relationships. By understanding attachment and trauma, the therapist can effectively work with challenging patients and get to the heart of the problem.

ACKNOWLEDGEMENTS

Foremost, I want to thank my family for all their support. A huge thanks to my friend and psychiatrist colleague Dr. Thanh Nguyen for his timely content editing of the entire book. This book was started with the encouragement and support from my friend and colleague Dr. Laurence Batmazian, who also provided editorial comments. I want to thank Dr. David Poon and Dr. Aaron Wu as well for reviewing the book and providing editorial comments. My interest in psychotherapy first began in medical school under the supervision of Dr. Carson Chrenek. I also want to thank Dr. Paula Ravitz, Dr. Yves Talbot, Dr. Kristina Powles, and Dr. Clare Pain for their inspirations and for expanding my psychotherapy knowledge. Dr. Michael Myers and Dr. Warren Rubenstein provided guidance and insights about the book publication process. Lastly, I want to thank the University of Toronto's Department of Family and Community Medicine for providing financial support through the Faculty Development Grant.

BIBLIOGRAPHY

Agras, W., & Robinson, A. (Ed.) (2017). *The Oxford Handbook of Eating Disorders, 2nd Edition.* Oxford University Press.

Akyuz, G., Kugu, N., Akyuz, A., & Dogan, O. (2004). "Dissociation and Childhood Abuse History in Epileptic and Pseudoseizure Patients." *Epileptic Disord.* Sep; 6(3):187-92.

Alberts, H. (2019). *3 Self-compassion Exercises for Helping Professionals.* Positive Psychology Program B.V. https://positivepsychology.com/wp-content/uploads/3-Self-Compassion-Exercises-Pack.pdf

American Psychiatric Association. (2022). *Diagnostic and Statistical Manual of Mental Disorders* (5th ed., text rev.). https://doi.org/10.1176/appi.books.9780890425787

American Society of Clinical Hypnosis. 2023. *About Hypnosis.* https://www.asch.net/aws/ASCH/pt/sp/about-hypnosis#h_7750676951516248446600672

Barlow, D. (2014). *Clinical Handbook of Psychological Disorders: A Step-by-step Treatment Manual* (5th ed.). The Guilford Press.

Bateman, A., & Fonagy, P. (2016). *Mentalization Based Treatment for Personality Disorders: A Practical Guide.* Oxford University Press.

Bleiberg, K., & Markowitz, J. (2019, March). "Interpersonal Psychotherapy for PTSD: Treating Trauma without Exposure." *Journal of Psychotherapy Integration.* 29(1), 15–22.

Bohus, M. (2019). *General Overview: Phases and Modules of DBT-PTSD.* University of Toronto.

Brown, B. (2018). *Dare to Lead: Brave Work. Tough Conversations. Whole Hearts.* Random House.

Brown, D. (2020, July 27-31). *31st Annual Summer Seminars: Complex Psychological Trauma and Recovery* [Course]. Harvard Medical School, Boston, MA, United States.

Cannon, G. (2020). *Clinical Hypnosis* [Course]. School of Continuing Studies, University of Toronto, Toronto, ON, Canada.

CaseyHouse. (2015, March). *Dr. Clare Pain—What's Traumatic about Trauma* [Video]. YouTube. https://www.youtube.com/watch?v=KfsOJoqY0RE

Clark, D., & Beck, A. (2011). *The Anxiety and Worry Workbook: The Cognitive Behavioral Solution.* The Guilford Press.

Craig, G. (2019, November). Official EFT Tutorial. The Gary Craig Official EFT Training Centers. https://emofree.com/english/eft-tutorial-en/eft-tapping-tutorial-en.html

Crawford, A., Adler Nevo, G., Cassin, S., & Segal, Z. (2021, January 5-March 30). *ECHO Ontario Psychotherapy Module 1: Cognitive Behavioural Therapy (CBT)* [Course]. ECHO Ontario Mental Health (ONMH), Toronto, ON, Canada.

Crawford, A., Lodenquai, G., Watson, P., Maunder, R., Boritz, T., Kirva, A., Clarkin, C., & Legary, E. (2021, April 20-June 22). *ECHO Ontario Psychotherapy- Developmental Trauma and Resilience* [Course]. ECHO Ontario Mental Health (ONMH), Toronto, ON, Canada.

Felitti, V., Anda, R., Nordenberg, D., et al. (1998). *Relationship of childhood abuse and household dysfunction to many of the leading causes of death in adults. The Adverse Childhood Experiences (ACE) Study.* Am J Prev Med. May;14(4):245-58. doi: 10.1016/s0749-3797(98)00017-8.

Fisher, R., & Ury, W. (2011). *Getting to Yes: Negotiating Agreement Without Giving In.* (B. Patton, Ed.). Penguin Books. (Original work published 1991).

Ford, J., & Courtois, C. (Ed.). (2020). *Treating Complex Traumatic Stress Disorders in Adults: Scientific Foundations and Therapeutic Models, Second Edition.* The Guilford Press.

Greenberger, D., & Padesky, C. (1995). *Mind Over Mood: Change How You Feel by Changing the Way You Think.* The Guilford Press.

Hall, K., Gibbie, T., & Lubman, D. (2012). *Motivational Interviewing Techniques: Facilitating Behaviour Change in the General Practice Setting.* Australian Family Physician. 41(9), 660–667.

Howell, E. (2011). *Understanding and Treating Dissociative Identity Disorder: A Relational Approach.* Routledge.

International Society for the Study of Trauma and Dissociation. (2023). *Resources.* https://www.isst-d.org/resources/

Kershaw, C., & Wade, B. (2017). *2-Day Hypnosis for Trauma & PTSD Certificate Course: A Hypnosis, Mind/Body & Neuroscience Approach to Effectively Treat Trauma & PTSD* [Course]. PESI, Eau Claire, WI, United States.

Kinsley, S. (2021, January 26-February 16). *Trauma-Informed Mindful Movement* [Course]. School of Continuing Studies, University of Toronto, Toronto, ON, Canada.

Kluft, R. (2012). "Hypnosis in the Treatment of Dissociative Identity Disorder and Allied States: an Overview and Case Study." *South African Journal of Psychology*, 42(2), 146–155. https://doi.org/10.1177/008124631204200202

Levine, B., Manly, T., Robertson I. (2012). *Goal Management Training Participant Workbook.* Baycrest.

Lillas, C., & Turnbull, J. (2008). *Infant Child Mental Health Early Technique and Relationship-based Therapies: A Neurorelational Framework for Interdisciplinary Practice.* Norton Professional Books.

Linehan, M. (2014). *DBT Skills Training Manual, Second Edition.* The Guilford Press.

Manber, R., & Carney, C. (2015). *Treatment Plans and Techniques for Insomnia: A Case Formulation Approach.* The Guilford Press.

Martin, S. (2019). *10 Ways to Build and Preserve Better Boundaries.* PsychCentral. https://psychcentral.com/lib/10-way-to-build-and-preserve-better-boundaries

Maves, P. (2020, November 6). *Integrative Techniques in the Treatment of Dissociative Identity Disorders (DID)* [Webinar]. ISSTD, Arlington, VA, United States.

Medical University of South Carolina. (2017). *TF-CBT Web 2.0: A Course for Trauma-Focused Cognitive Behavioral Therapy.* https://tfcbt2.musc.edu/en

Muller, R. (2018). *Trauma and the Struggle to Open Up: From Avoidance to Recovery and Growth.* Norton Professional Books.

Myers, M. (2020). *Becoming a Doctors' Doctor: A Memoir.* Independently Published.

Myers, M. (2017). *Why Physicians Die by Suicide: Lessons Learned from Their Families and Others Who Cared.* Independently Published.

Nash, Jo. (2015, February 12). *The 5 Founding Fathers and A History of Positive Psychology.* https://positivepsychology.com/founding-fathers/

National Institute for the Clinical Application of Behavioral Medicine. (2023). *The Treating Trauma*

Master Series: A 5-Module Series on the Treatment of Trauma. https://www.nicabm.com/program/treating-trauma-master/?del=gad.1.sitelink.ttms&network=g&utm_source=google&utm_medium=cpc&utm_campaign=9310101522&ad_group_id=93592120225&utm_term=%2Bnicabm&utm_content=417451850131&gclid=EAIaIQobChMIot-A1N-t_wIVpNvjBx3xXg45EAAYASABEgLHCvD_BwE

Ogden, P., & Fisher, J. (2015). *Sensorimotor Psychotherapy: Techniques for Trauma and Attachment.* Norton Professional Books.

Ogden, P., Minton, K., & Pain, C. (2006). *Trauma and the Body: A Sensorimotor Approach to Psychotherapy.* Norton Professional Books.

Ravitz, P., Maunder, R., et al. (2015). *Psychotherapy Essentials To Go 6 Book Set.* Norton Professional Books.

Richter, P. Taube-Schiff, M., Grapko, D., et al. (2021, September 23-November 25). *CBT for Obsessive Compulsive Disorder* [Course]. ECHO Ontario Mental Health (ONMH), Toronto, ON, Canada.

Robertson, S., & Zambrano, D. (2023, March 29-April 19). *Finding Your Edge: Mindfulness and Optimal Performance* [Course]. School of Continuing Studies, University of Toronto, Toronto, ON, Canada.

Schwartz, R., & Sweezy, M. (2019). *Internal Family Systems Therapy, Second Edition.* The Guilford Press.

The Gatehouse. (2020, May). *Phase 1 Peer Support Group Program Participant Manual.* https://thegatehouse.org

The National Health Service. (2022, November 10). *Overview - Cognitive behavioural therapy (CBT).* https://www.nhs.uk/mental-health/

talking-therapies-medicine-treatments/talking-therapies-and-counselling/cognitive-behavioural-therapy-cbt/overview/

Therapist Aid. (2021). *Body Image Discussion Questions.* https://www.therapistaid.com/worksheets/body-image-discussion-questions

Toneatto, T. (2021, February 20-28). *Clinical Applications of Buddhist Psychology* [Course]. School of Continuing Studies, University of Toronto, Toronto, ON, Canada.

United States Department of Veterans Affairs. (2013). *PFA Mobile Psychological First Aid.* https://www.ptsd.va.gov/appvid/mobile/pfa_app_pro.asp

United States Department of Veterans Affairs. (2023, May). *PTSD: National Center for PTSD.* https://www.ptsd.va.gov/

Van der Kolk, B. (2020, October 8-9). *The Body Keeps Score—Trauma Healing with Bessel van der Kolk, MD* [Conference presentation]. PESI 2-Day: Trauma Conference, Boston, MA, United States.

Young, J., & Brown, G. (2003). *Young Schema Questionnaire (YSQ-L3).* Psychology Training. https://psychology-training.com.au/wp-content/uploads/2017/04/Young-Schema-Questionnaire-L3.pdf

ACRONYM INDEX

ACEs: Adverse Childhood Experiences

ACT: Acceptance and Commitment Therapy

ADHD: Attention Deficit Hyperactivity Disorder

BPD: Borderline Personality Disorder

CBT: Cognitive Behavioural Therapy

CPT: Cognitive Processing Therapy

cPTSD: Complex PTSD

CT: Complex Trauma

DBT: Dialectical Behaviour Therapy

DSM: Diagnostic and Statistical Manual of Mental Disorders

DTD: Developmental Trauma Disorder

EMDR: Eye Movement Desensitization and Reprocessing

GAD: Generalized Anxiety Disorder

IBS: Irritable Bowel Syndrome

IPT: Interpersonal Therapy

OCD: Obsessive-compulsive Disorder

PTSD: Post-traumatic Stress Disorder

PVD: Peripheral Vascular Disease

Printed in Canada